The **Volumetrics**
Eating
Plan

Also by Barbara Rolls, Ph.D.

The Volumetrics Weight-Control Plan

Techniques and

Recipes for

Feeling Full

on Fewer Calories

The
Volumetrics
Eating
Plan

Barbara Rolls, Ph.D.

HarperCollins*Publishers*

HarperCollins books may be purchased for educational, business, or sales promotional use. For information, please write: Special Markets Department, HarperCollins Publishers Inc., 10 East 53rd Street, New York, NY 10022.

FIRST EDITION

Designed by Laura Lindgren and Jessica Shatan

Printed on acid-free paper

Library of Congress Cataloging-in-Publication Data

Rolls, Barbara J.
    The volumetrics eating plan : techniques and recipes for feeling full on fewer calories / Barbara Rolls.—1st ed.
        p.   cm.
    Includes bibliographical references and index.
    ISBN 0-06-073729-8 (alk. paper)
    1. Reducing diets—Recipes.   2. Appetite.   3. Food—Caloric content.   I. Title.
    RM222.2.R6275 2005   2004054045
    641.5'635—dc22

05   06   07   08   09   DIX/RRD   10   9   8   7   6   5   4   3   2   1

To my dad, Howard Simons

who, along with my mom, Patricia,

taught me the importance of healthy eating.

◆　◆　◆

Also for my daughters,

Melissa and Juliet,

who continue to make me proud.

Contents

Acknowledgments ix

1 • **Welcome to Volumetrics** 1

2 • **Your Personal Weight Management Plan** 31

3 • **Breakfast** 59

Jennifer's Fruit-Smothered Whole-Wheat Buttermilk Pancakes 62
Baked Berry French Toast 64
Mexican Egg Wrap 65
Piquant Frittata 66
Blueberry Applesauce Muffins 68
Creamy Apricot Oatmeal 69

4 • **Appetizers, Starters, and Snacks** 71

Vegetable Party Platter 74
House Dressing 76
Mel's Fresh Lemon Hummus 77
Tex-Mex Salsa 78
White Bean Bruschetta 79
Lemon Shrimp Bruschetta 80
Insalata Caprese 81
Asian Spring Rolls with Soy-Ginger Dipping Sauce 82
Sesame Mushroom Kebobs 84
Mushroom and Cheese Quesadillas with Mango Salsa 85

Stuffed Mushrooms Florentine 86
Guacamole 88
Mango Salsa 88
Yogurt Cheese 89
B's Favorite Smoothie 90
Tropical Island Smoothie 91

5 • **Soups** 93

Corn and Tomato Chowder 95
Autumn Harvest Pumpkin Soup 96
Creamy Broccoli Soup 98
Curried Cauliflower Soup 100
Rustic Tomato Soup 101
Minestrone 102
Asian Black Bean Soup 104
Cannellini Bean Soup 105
Lentil and Tomato Soup 106
Vegetarian Barley Soup 107
Hearty Chicken and Vegetable Soup 108
Gazpacho 110

6 • **Sandwiches and Wraps** 111

Almond Chicken Salad Sandwich 114
Cold-Cut Combo Sandwich 116
Mediterranean Turkey Sandwich 117
Open-Faced Roast Beef Sandwich 118
Roasted Portobello Sandwich 119
Buffalo Chicken Wraps 120

Asian Chicken Wraps 122

Chicken and Avocado Pita
  Pockets 123

Zesty Tuna Salad Pita 124

All American Hamburger 126

7 • Salads and Salad Dressings 127

Charlie's Greek Salad 130

Creamy Cucumber and Dill
  Salad 132

Fennel, Orange, and Arugula
  Salad 133

Volumetrics Salad 134

Lemony Fennel Salad 136

Insalata Mista 137

Fresh Fruit and Spinach Salad with
  Orange–Poppy Seed Dressing 138

Tangy Cole Slaw 139

Pepper Slaw 140

Thai Chicken Salad 142

California Cobb Salad with Nonfat
  Tomato and Herb Dressing 143

Santa Fe Steak Salad with Lime-
  Cilantro Dressing 144

Liz's Pasta Salad 146

Tabbouleh 148

Potato Salad with Green Beans and
  Tarragon 149

Tuna and White Bean Salad 150

Balsamic Dressing 152

Dijon Vinaigrette 152

Citrus-Ginger Dressing 153

Italian Dressing 153

8 • Vegetables and Vegetarian Dishes 155

Minted Broccoli 158

Garlic-Roasted Vegetables 160

Ratatouille 162

Roasted Asparagus 163

Stir-Fried Green Beans 164

Crisp Stir-Fried Vegetables 166

Tofu Pad Thai 167

New Potatoes with Peas 168

Oven-Roasted Potatoes 169

Smashed Potatoes 170

Herbed Barley Stuffed Squash 171

Bulgur and Vegetable Stuffed
  Peppers 172

Chickpea Curry 174

Eggplant "Lasagna" 175

Classic Vegetarian Vegetable
  Stew 176

9 • Meats 179

Stir-Fried Beef with Snow Peas
  and Tomatoes 181

Old World Goulash 182

Shepherd's Pie 184

Nouveau Lamb Stew 186

Pork Chops with Orange-Soy
  Sauce 188

Roasted Lamb Chops with
    Gremolata 190

10 · **Fish and Shellfish** 191

Poach-Roast Salmon with Yogurt
    and Dill Sauce 193
Baked Tilapia with Sautéed
    Vegetables 194
Sautéed Flounder with
    Lemon Sauce 196
Fillet of Sole and Vegetable
    Parcels 197
Jenny's Caribbean Tuna and Fruit
    Kebobs 198
Shrimp Creole 199
Shrimp Fried Rice 200
Fiesta Fish Stew 202

11 · **Poultry** 203

Chicken Parmesan 205
Chicken Merlot 206
South of the Border Chicken
    Stew 208
Chicken Provençal 210
Stir-Fried Turkey with Crunchy
    Vegetables 211
Italian Turkey Spirals 212

12 · **Beans, Rice, and Grains** 213

Garden Chili 216
Bayou Red Beans and Rice 218
Paella Sencillo 220
Vegetable Pilaf 221
Risotto Primavera 222
Mary's Quinoa with Lime 224

13 · **Pasta and Pizza** 225

Charlie's Pasta Primavera 228
Oceanside Pasta 230
Penne with Olives and Spinach 232
Spaghetti with Tomato and Fresh
    Basil Sauce 233
Veggie-Stuffed Macaroni and
    Cheese 234
Broccoli and Tomato Stuffed
    Shells 236
The Aristotle Pizza 237
Garden-Fresh Vegetable Pizza 238
Pizza Margherita 239
Chicken Fajita Pizza 240
Turkey-Pepperoni Pizza 242

14 · **Desserts and Fruit** 243

Balsamic Berries 246
Grilled Banana Splits 248
Four-Fruit Compote 249
Ruby-Red Poached Pears with
    Raspberry Sauce 250
Fresh Fruit Parfait 252
Raspberry-Apple Crumble 254
Raspberry-Topped Ricotta Cakes 255
Strawberry Trifle with Lemon
    Cream 256
Maple Crème Caramel 258
Chocolate Fondue with Fresh Fruit 259

15 · **Your Personal
    Eating Plan** 261

Resources 293
References 297
Index 301
Conversion Chart 317

Acknowledgments

First and foremost I want to thank my partner, Charlie Brueggebors, whose creative cooking and organizational skills made this book possible. He developed and tested many of the recipes, and was happy to share all that he has learned over the years about making recipes both delicious and volumetric. Members of my lab, Jenny Ledikwe, Jennifer Meengs, and Anne Gooch, helped him. They have not only spent many evenings and weekends testing Charlie's recipes, but have also gladly shared some of their own favorites. Jenny has worked diligently putting together charts and helping me with the overall organization of the book. Julie Ello-Martin, one of my doctoral students, developed some of the key messages related to energy density and weight loss. Elizabeth Bell and Julie Flood provided insightful comments on the manuscript.

Michael Black of Black Sun Studio, L.L.C. expertly photographed the food with the assistance of food stylist Kerri Kinzle Rossi. They worked tirelessly to illustrate the principles of *Volumetrics* in the straightforward and elegant photos included here.

I am grateful for all of the advice and wisdom that my agent, Alice Martell of The Martell Agency, has provided. I thank my editor, Susan Friedland, for continuing to have the vision to support *Volumetrics*—her insights as to how to communicate key messages have been invaluable. Her assistant, Califia Suntree, has expertly helped with many practical issues.

I want to thank the many people who contributed recipe suggestions, and the readers of *The Volumetrics Weight-Control Plan* who took time to share their experiences when following *Volumetrics*. Their enthusiasm was my inspiration for this book.

Without my students, staff, and colleagues at Penn State who, over the years, have helped conceive and conduct our studies, the science to support this plan would not be there. I thank them and all of the study participants who have volunteered to let us study their eating behavior. I am extremely grateful to the National Institute of Diabetes and Digestive and Kidney Diseases for funding my research.

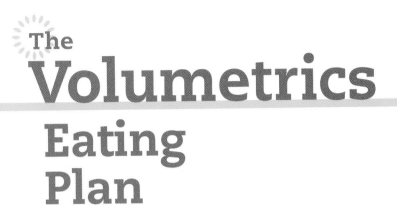

The Volumetrics Eating Plan

1 Welcome to Volumetrics

Fed up with fad diets that ask you to give up your favorite foods? Tired of feeling ravenous when cutting back on calories? Searching for a sensible, healthy way to manage your weight? Welcome to *Volumetrics*! With this weight management plan, you'll learn how to fit your favorite foods into your day while eating nutritiously. Perhaps the best news of all is that you'll discover why eating more, not less, of certain foods can be the answer to losing weight and keeping it off.

I am not going to promise that managing your weight will be easy, but I will show you how to make it healthy and sustainable. If you have found that your weight has been creeping up over the years, you are certainly not alone. More than half of all adults in America are overweight or obese. We are surrounded by a huge variety of tempting high-calorie foods, and we are less and less active. For most of us, it is difficult to avoid putting on weight in this *obesigenic* environment. To resist the almost inevitable weight gain over time, you need sound strategies. I will show you what recent research reveals about how to choose foods that will help you to maintain or reach your optimal weight.

First, let me share with you some information about why I am qualified to help direct your food choices. I have spent my career studying eating behavior and weight management. As a professor of nutritional sciences at Penn State University, I train students and conduct research funded by the National Institutes of Health. My lab includes a large research kitchen and dining area. For our studies, people come to the dining area to eat. We test how different properties of foods such as calorie density, fat content, or portion size affect how much people eat, how hungry they feel, and what affects the enjoyment of the foods being eaten. Our studies have led to a better understanding of which foods can help curb hunger without adding extra calories. It is exciting to be doing work that has an impact on the biggest health challenge we have ever faced as a nation—the obesity epidemic. This book gives me the opportunity to take what we have learned in the laboratory and translate it into a sensible, easy-to-follow eating plan that you can use. I look forward to telling you about the basics of healthy weight management.

Volumetrics is an eating plan based on the latest research on how to control hunger while managing calories to lose weight or to hold steady at your current weight. The plan also helps ensure that you are eating a balanced and nutritious diet. Often, when people decide to make the commitment to lose weight, they forget that the foods they eat affect a lot more than their weight. When you are eating fewer calories than you normally do, it is more important than ever to eat a good balance of nutrients. Because you are eating less, you are already at higher risk of not getting an adequate amount of key nutrients. Dieting is the worst possible time to cut out entire food groups. Although *Volumetrics* can be used to help achieve your goal weight, it is not just for those who want to manage their weight. Since it is a practical guide to nutritious and satisfying foods, it will help to establish habits associated with eating well for optimal health.

Weight-loss clinics across the country are using *Volumetrics*. Both physicians and dietitians love it because it is a healthy, sensible weight management program. They tell me that their patients are asking for simple and practical advice, as well as recipes to help them achieve and sustain their weight loss. This book will give you just that. It is intended as a companion to *The Volumetrics Weight-Control Plan*. You can read more about the science behind Volumetrics in that book.

This book is filled with simple tips on how you can enjoy delicious food while managing your weight. After being introduced to the basics of *Volumetrics* in this chapter, you will develop your personalized weight management plan in Chapter 2. A big challenge for me has been to show you how to fit *Volumetrics* into your busy life. I know when I come home from a day at work, I don't want to spend a lot of time in the kitchen. In Chapters 3 to 14, you will find recipes for tasty, easy-to-prepare dishes. In addition to the recipes, I give you a variety of tools to help you follow *The Volumetrics Eating Plan:*

- Techniques for modifying your favorite recipes and incorporating more volumetric foods into your diet.
- A menu plan to give you structure as you learn about what and how much you should be eating. If you find it helpful, you can continue to use this plan—personalize it to suit your preferences.
- A variety of quick meal ideas in the menu plan.
- Modular lists of foods that are equivalent in calories to help you add variety to your menus.
- Self-monitoring charts to keep you on track.

For those of you who like structure, I have included a menu plan in Chapter 15 to guide you through your first month of *Volumetrics* eating. In the long run, I want to teach you the principles of healthy eating for weight management, so you can apply them no matter the situation. I will show you how to find an eating pattern that is so enjoyable that you will want to sustain it. I can assure you that, if you eat the Volumetrics way, you will be eating a diet that fits with the recommendations of the major health organizations in America and that will help you to lose weight or keep extra pounds from sneaking up on you.

The Volumetrics Eating Plan

- Focuses on what you can eat, not on what you must give up.
- Is based on sound nutritional advice widely accepted by health professionals.
- Emphasizes that the only proven way to lose weight is to eat fewer calories than your body uses as fuel for your activities.
- Stresses that when you are managing calories it is more important than ever to eat a good balance of foods and nutrients.
- Teaches you to make food choices that will help control hunger and enhance satiety.
- Shows you how to fit your favorite foods into your diet.
- Reinforces eating and activity patterns that you can sustain for a lifetime of achieving your own healthy weight.

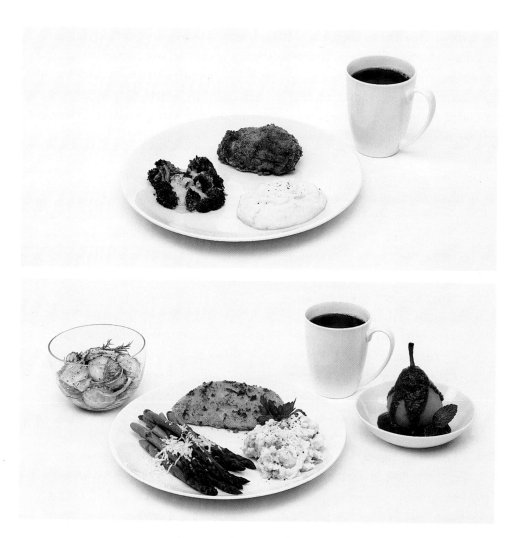

Both of these meals contain 500 calories. Yes, that is right; they both contain the same number of calories! The traditional meal in the top photo gives you only small portions of fried chicken, mashed potatoes, and cheesy broccoli. The large meal in the bottom photo is based on the principles of *Volumetrics*. This volumetric meal is reduced in fat, high in fruits and veggies, and full of flavor. It contains Creamy Cucumber and Dill Salad (page 132), Chicken Parmesan (page 205), Smashed Potatoes (page 170), Roasted Asparagus (page 163), and a Ruby-Red Poached Pears with Raspberry Sauce (page 250). Which meal would you find to be more satisfying?

Many people have contacted me to share their Volumetrics' success stories, including Jill O'Nan. Testimonials don't prove that a diet will work for everybody, but they can certainly be inspiring. Jill, a professional writer, contacted me after her first six months following *Volumetrics* and has kept in touch for several years now. I want to share her story with you to show you the impact that eating a nutritious volumetric diet can have on hunger and weight.

At 360 pounds, I made a startling discovery—I was underfed! Not in terms of calories, of course, but in terms of volume. A lifelong lover of fast food, my usual lunch was a burger and fries. By midafternoon I was hungry again, and found myself snacking on cookies, candy, and crackers to tide me over. The frozen dinners I ate were small, 300-calorie ones, which I typically topped off with ice cream because I was still hungry. In fact, hunger was a constant fact of life for me, whether I was trying to diet or not.

The Volumetrics Weight-Control Plan showed me how to change that by explaining the relationship between calories, volume, and satiety. As a morbidly obese person, it had never occurred to me that I should be eating more. But as I read the book, I realized that, indeed, the amount of food I ate every day was not satisfying, and my constant hunger was causing me to make increasingly poor food choices. The message that I could lose weight while feeling full was unique and compelling: No other diet addressed the importance of satiety (except to imply that dieters should be prepared to suffer as penance for having overeaten in the first place)!

I began my Volumetrics weight-control plan in April 2001. The key for me was learning how to become a "calorie bargain hunter." High-energy-dense foods like French fries and ice cream, I soon realized, were not going to be part of my daily food plan. The calories were too high and the servings too small. Large servings of low-energy-dense foods like fruit, vegetables, and soups, however, were bona fide bargains, offering high satisfaction and nutrition at a low calorie cost. I began shopping for quality produce and substituted soups, salads and vegetables for the starchy side dishes I'd eaten before. Nonfat yogurt and fruit took the place of ice cream for dessert. I even traded in my beloved hamburgers for leaner proteins like chicken and fish.

My calorie bargain hunting paid off. While my meals got bigger, I got smaller—176 pounds smaller as of this writing. By applying volumetric principles, I can manage my food intake, maintain a feeling of satiety, and continue to meet my weight-loss goals. And that's the most satisfying feeling of all.

SATIETY—THE MISSING INGREDIENT

Any diet that helps you cut calories will help you lose weight. Some people find it easy to reduce fat, while others don't mind limiting carbohydrates—at least in the short term. The problem is that most of us cannot imagine life without chocolate and ice cream, or pasta, bread, and potatoes. Cutting out or drastically restricting foods is simply not sustainable. And when you do give in and eat the banned foods, you feel guilty. I am going to show you how to get rid of the guilt and fit every kind of food into your diet. Of course, some foods need to be approached with more moderation than others!

Many diets tell you that simply by choosing particular foods or combinations of nutrients your body will eliminate excess calories and burn off body fat. Believe me, if there were such a magic metabolic solution, those of us who spend our lives researching ways to battle the epidemic of obesity would be the first to tell you about it. The truth is that you must eat fewer calories to lose weight and, when you do that, your body uses all of the food you eat for energy, regardless of whether it is primarily carbohydrates, fat, or protein. While there are some differences in how your body uses the different nutrients as fuel, these have only a small effect on your body weight.

The foods and nutrients you choose do make a difference to how well you will be able to sustain a diet. Not only do you need to choose foods that are nutritious and enjoyable, you should make selections that will keep hunger at bay. *Volumetrics* is based on the science of *satiety,* the feeling of fullness and satisfaction that you should have at the end of a meal.

Satiety is the missing ingredient in weight management. If you limit calories by simply eating less, you'll feel hungry and deprived. You may be able to stick to such a diet for the short term, but to be successful at lifelong weight management, you'll need to make food choices that help you feel full with fewer calories. For any given level of calories, some foods keep you full and satisfied until the next meal, while with others hunger returns soon after eating. I am going to show you how to make the right food choices to control hunger so you can lose weight, keep it off, and stay healthy. Feeling full and satisfied while eating foods you like is a critical part of this eating plan.

You can choose "high-satiety food." The basics are simple:

- Eat foods low in energy density.
- Choose foods high in fiber.
- Eat adequate amounts of lean protein.
- Reduce intake of fat.

Let me tell you about these properties of food that affect satiety.

The food label and satiety

You will be learning how you can use *energy density* (calories per gram), fiber, protein, and fat to make more satiating food choices. Let's take a look at the Nutrition Facts information on a food label to find out where these are listed. Remember, these values are the amount in *one* serving and there may be more than one serving in a package! I'll show you how to use the Nutrition Facts label to calculate energy density later (page 18).

Nutrition Facts		
Serving Size 1 cup (253g)		← Grams
Servings Per Container 4		← Number of Servings
Amount Per Serving		
Calories → **Calories** 260	Calories from Fat 72	
	% Daily Value*	
Fat → **Total Fat** 8g	13%	
Saturated Fat 3g	17%	
Cholesterol 130mg	44%	
Sodium 1010mg	42%	
Total Carbohydrate 22g	7%	
Fiber → Dietary Fiber 9g	36%	
Sugars 4g		
Protein → **Protein** 25g		

ENERGY DENSITY (E.D.)

When trying to consume fewer calories, you should be aware of the amount of calories in a given weight of food (calories per gram). A food that is high in energy density (or calorie density) provides a large amount of calories in a small weight, while a food of low energy density has fewer calories for the same amount (weight). With foods of lower energy density, you can eat a larger portion (weight) for the same calories. To enhance satiety, you want to choose foods that contain the smallest number of calories in the biggest portion—these are foods low in energy density.

Why does this matter? Research shows that, over a day or two, a person will eat about the same weight of food. Obviously, there is some variability—on days that someone eats out, for example, she may eat more food. But, in general, when scientists have looked at what people report they eat, or when food intake has been measured in the lab, the weight of food a person eats is more similar from day to day than the number of calories consumed. It seems that we have learned how much food it takes to satisfy our hunger, and that is what we choose to eat. In my lab, we have conducted a number of studies showing that people help themselves to equal amounts of similar foods regardless of the calorie content. Therefore, when the energy density of a food, such as a casserole, is reduced by adding water or water-rich vegetables, people eat the same amount of food and, as a result, they eat fewer calories. Significantly, they feel just as full and satisfied. I will tell you more about our studies on energy density and satiety in later chapters. You can also read about them in The *Volumetrics Weight-Control Plan.*

The takeaway message from these studies is that by choosing foods that have fewer calories in your usual weight of food, you will end up eating fewer calories. And you won't feel any hungrier! I am going to give you lots of tips as to how to lower the energy density of your diet so that you can eat a satisfying amount of food while losing weight. For example, you'll learn how to lower the energy density of macaroni and cheese, a popular food in many households. For the same calories you can have a much larger portion, almost twice as much, of the Veggie-Stuffed Macaroni and Cheese (page 234), compared to a traditional macaroni-and-cheese recipe.

Adding water-rich ingredients such as vegetables lowers the energy density. Cutting out some of the fat can also lower it. Fat is the most energy-dense component of food. It really packs the calories into food, providing 9 calories per gram, more than twice as many as carbohydrates or protein, which provide 4 calories per gram. This high energy density makes fat calories easy to overeat. In general, if you lower the fat content of a food, you will get a bigger portion for the same number of calories. Think about it—if you leave the butter off your bread, you can have two slices instead of the one buttered slice for the same 140 calories. If you choose skim milk rather than whole milk, you will get almost twice as much for the same calories. I'll discuss fat reduction strategies in more detail on pages 13–16.

While fat has a big impact on energy density, water has an even greater effect. Water has an energy density of 0. It has weight but no calories at all! Foods with a high water content influence satiety because water dilutes the calories in food, adding weight and volume without adding calories. If you choose water-rich foods, you can have satisfying portions with few calories. Consider grapes compared to raisins. They are the same food, but removing the water drastically affects how much you can eat. In a 100 calorie snack, you get only ¼ cup of raisins compared to 2 cups of grapes.

Where the calories are

To understand where the calories are in your food, imagine that each of the scale weights is a 1-gram weight (there are 28 grams in an ounce). Each dot represents one calorie. The number of dots shows the energy (or calorie) density of the major components of the foods you eat. As you can see, the energy density varies widely, from 9 calories per gram (cal/g) for fat, 7 for alcohol, 4 for carbohydrate and protein, 2 for fiber, to 0 for water. Remember that low-energy-dense foods with few calories per gram give you bigger, more satisfying portions than high-energy-dense foods.

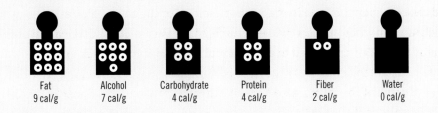

| Fat | Alcohol | Carbohydrate | Protein | Fiber | Water |
| 9 cal/g | 7 cal/g | 4 cal/g | 4 cal/g | 2 cal/g | 0 cal/g |

The water content of foods

There are huge differences in the water content of foods. Choose foods that have high water content and you will feel full on fewer calories.

Food	Water Content (percent)
Fruits and vegetables	80–95
Soups	80–95
Hot cereal	85
Yogurt, low-fat fruit, flavored	75
Egg, boiled	75
Pasta, cooked	65
Fish and seafood	60–85
Meats	45–65
Bread	35–40
Cheese	35
Nuts	2–5
Saltine crackers	3
Potato chips	2
Oil	0

Don't think that you can simply drink lots of water—this is healthy, but it won't fill you up. You'll need to eat more foods that are naturally rich in water, such as fruits, vegetables, low-fat milk, and cooked grains. You should also be eating more water-rich dishes: soups, stews, casseroles, pasta with vegetables, and fruit-based desserts. But you'll have to limit the portion size and frequency of foods that are low in water, such as high-fat foods like potato chips, as well as low-fat and fat-free foods that contain little moisture, like pretzels, crackers, and fat-free cookies.

Throughout the book I am going to show you how to lower the energy density of a wide variety of dishes. The recipes that I chose include many favorite foods such as pancakes (page 62), pasta salad (page 146), and even pepperoni pizza (page 242). I have ensured that they are all delicious and satisfying.

FIBER AND OTHER CARBOHYDRATES

Grains, breads, cereals, vegetables, fruits, and refined sugar contain primarily carbo-hydrates, which serve as the body's main fuel. This broad range of foods provides more than half of the calories most of us consume. You don't have to eliminate car-bohydrates from your diet to lose weight—to do so would mean you would miss out on valuable nutrients. Instead, choose wisely—go for the carbohydrate-containing foods that provide the most nutrients and the most satiety. Choose those high in water and fiber, particularly vegetables, fruits, and whole grains.

Fiber is a form of carbohydrate that cannot be fully digested. Because it has so few calories that your body can use (1.5 to 2.5 per gram) compared to other nutrients, the addition of fiber helps to reduce the energy density of foods. However, since only small amounts can be added to most foods, fiber's impact on energy density is less than that of water. Fiber has been shown to increase satiety not only by lowering the energy density of foods but also by slowing the rate that foods pass through the di-gestive system. Most people fall far short of the recommended fiber intake, which is 25 grams a day for women and 38 grams for men. Choosing fiber-rich foods can help you to lose weight while eating nutritious foods. Simply doubling the amount of fiber you eat from the average of 15 grams per day to around 30 grams helps reduce calorie intake. Even better for those of you wanting to lose weight is that studies have shown that, in just four months, this increased fiber intake resulted in the

Where to find the fiber

- Always think about how you can add vegetables and fruits to meals and snacks.
- Eat fruits and vegetables whole, peeling only when necessary.
- Find the whole grains—look in breads and cereal.
  - Check the label. You are looking for breads that are 100 percent whole-wheat or grain or that list the whole grains first in the ingredients. Look for at least 2 grams of fiber per slice.
  - Choose breakfast cereals wisely. For healthy fast food in a box, find high-fiber cereals you enjoy. Select cereals that have at least 3 grams of fiber per serving.
  - Choose brown rice and whole-wheat or wheat-blend pasta.
- Look for legumes such as kidney beans or black beans, lentils, chickpeas, and split peas; which are loaded with fiber.
  - Add these to pastas, soups, and stews.
  - Cook them and add to burgers and meat loaf.

consumption of fewer calories, which led to an average weight loss of five pounds—with no dieting!

Generally, whole foods, rather than those that have been processed, are good choices. Processing can destroy or remove the fiber from foods so they provide less satiety. For example, whole fruit is more satiating than juice, which contains very little fiber. Look for whole grains, as they are nutritious and require more chewing, which slows eating and provides lots of sensory satisfaction. Just a few of the fiber-rich volumetric recipes you'll discover include Creamy Apricot Oatmeal (page 69), Asian Black Bean Soup (page 104), Bayou Red Beans and Rice (page 218), and Bulgur and Vegetable Stuffed Peppers (page 172).

PROTEIN FOR WEIGHT LOSS

You probably have heard a lot about higher-protein, lower-carbohydrate diets and weight loss in recent years. Some people say they find it easy to stick to these diets, at least for a while. This may be because high-protein foods can decrease hunger and prolong satiety more than foods high in either carbohydrate or fat. Eating enough protein-rich foods of low energy density is a good strategy for increasing satiety, especially if you are trying to lose weight. But eating more protein than your body needs is not going to boost your metabolism, build more muscle, or make you thinner! When you cut calories, you should make sure you are eating an adequate amount of protein and that your sources of protein are low in fat. The amount of protein you need each day is based on your body weight. The usual recommendation is 0.4 grams per pound body weight. If you are very active, you can go up to 0.8 grams per pound.

Tips for choosing high-protein foods wisely

- Choose moderate portions of lean protein-rich poultry, seafood, low-fat dairy foods, egg whites, tofu, and legumes, which are fairly low in energy density; combine them with low-energy-dense whole grains, vegetables, and fruits.
- Make sure there is a good source of low-fat protein at most meals. It could be non-fat milk with your cereal, water-packed tuna for lunch, or chicken or legumes for dinner.
- Find some low-calorie higher-protein snacks that you enjoy: yogurt, lean turkey slices, low-fat mozzarella sticks, or black bean dip or hummus served with veggies.
- When choosing meat, eliminate excess fat by removing the skin from poultry and trimming visible fat from lamb, beef, and pork.
- Egg whites contain no fat and may be eaten often. In many recipes, you can substitute two egg whites for one whole egg.

FINDING FLAVOR WITH LESS FAT

Fat adds delicious textures and carries the flavors in many of our favorite foods, so trying to give up all of the fat in your diet is not a palatable long-term solution to cutting calories. Plus, some fats are healthy, such as those in fish, nuts, avocados, and olives. You need to remind yourself that decreasing the amount of fat you eat will lower the energy density of your diet. In general, the lower the fat, the bigger the portion you get for the same number of calories. You need to find a level of fat in your food that helps you to lower the energy density, but still gives you enjoyment.

Once you learn to identify the sources of fat in your diet, there are many simple steps you can take to eat less without sacrificing taste. Check the Nutrition Facts label on food packages, looking at the number of fat grams per serving (page 7) and for fat-related packaging claims. About 20 to 30 percent of your calories should come from fat, which is 36 to 53 grams of fat per day if you are eating 1600 calories per day. An easy way to reduce your total fat intake is to eat more reduced-fat and low-fat foods and fewer high-fat foods. Foods specifically labeled low-fat have 3 grams or less of fat per serving, while those labeled reduced-fat or less fat have at least 25 percent less fat per serving than the food to which it is being compared.

Finding tasty reduced-fat foods is easier than ever before. Not only are there more products on the market than in the past, but also they are continually being improved, so they taste more like the full-fat foods. Make sure that you choose reduced-fat foods that are also lower in calories and energy density than their original version—check labels to compare calories. Try some of the new reduced-fat products—salad dressings are popular and even reduced-fat cheese has improved over the early rubbery versions. If you like them, use them to replace the higher fat options. This way you will be able to eat satisfying portions and keep your fat and calories under control.

While it is important to choose reduced-fat foods, you should keep in mind that not all fats are the same. Different types of fat have different effects on your health. You may have heard of *monounsaturated* fat, the type of fat found in fish, olives, nuts, and avocados. Monounsaturated fats, especially the omega-3 fatty acids found in fish, provide important health benefits, and may help reduce your risk of heart disease. You should enjoy moderate portions of foods containing monounsaturated fats. Remember that all fats are similar in energy density, so all are easy to overeat.

You should avoid saturated fats and transfats—they can raise your blood cholesterol levels and increase your risk of heart disease. Saturated fats are found in red meat and full-fat fat dairy products; transfats, often referred to as *partially hydrogenated oils,* are found in many commercial baked goods and fried foods. Limiting your intake of saturated fat and transfat not only helps you lower the energy density of your diet, but can also help improve your cardiovascular health.

Fat reduction strategies

Substitute reduced-fat or low-fat items for high-fat items

- Choose nonfat, low-fat, or reduced-fat spreads and dressings.
- Select broth-based soups rather than cream-based soups. Or, if you like creamy soups, make your own volumetrics soups such as Creamy Broccoli Soup (page 98) and Autumn Harvest Pumpkin Soup (page 96).
- Top a baked potato with nonfat or low-fat yogurt or sour cream, or Tex-Mex Salsa (page 78) instead of butter or full-fat sour cream.

Use alternative food items to flavor food when cooking

- Sauté mushrooms, onions, garlic, celery, and other veggies in bouillon, low-fat chicken stock, wine, or seasoned water instead of butter, margarine, or oil.
- Season your food with vegetables. Diced onion, garlic, celery, and bell pepper add flavor to many recipes.
- Enhance the taste of your foods with nonfat sauces and condiments such as ketchup, mustard, salsa, soy sauce, sweet-and-sour sauce, hot-pepper sauce, teriyaki sauce, fresh ginger, horseradish, vinegar, and Worcestershire sauce.
- Experiment with creative ways to add flavor to your foods without adding fat. For example, you can try lemon zest on rice, lime juice on fish, orange juice on pork, tomato salsa on baked chicken, or mustard on beef and chicken.
- Use herbs and spices.

Use alternative cooking methods

- Use cooking methods that are lower in added fat: baking, broiling, roasting, microwaving, steaming, and grilling.
- Use nonstick pans and skillets.
- Switch to cooking sprays in place of butter, margarine, or oil.
- Lightly stir-fry or sauté in small amounts of olive or canola oil or reduced-sodium broth.

Obvious ways to reduce the amount of oils, high-fat spreads, dressings, and sauces in your diet are to simply eat fewer of these foods or to eat them less often. Use these foods when it really matters to you—avoid using them out of habit. For example, if you dislike tossed salad without dressing, use only the amount of dressing necessary to give it a pleasant taste. On the other hand, if you can eat your dinner roll plain instead of simply spreading butter on it out of habit, break that habit and save those fat grams for foods that are more important to you. There will be more fat-saving tips throughout the book. For example, you'll learn how to make a delicious Risotto Primavera (page 222) that is much lower in fat than traditional risotto.

UNDERSTANDING ENERGY DENSITY AND FOOD CHOICES

Now that you understand that your food choices can affect satiety, it is time to show you how to use energy density to make food choices that will keep hunger under control. Remember, energy density is simply the calories in a fixed weight of food. I give you energy-density values as calories per gram rather than per ounce. Although you are probably more familiar with ounces, it is easier to understand energy density in terms of grams. If you look at a food label, you will see that portions are given in grams. From the label, I will show you how to easily calculate the number of calories per gram. To help you think about foods in terms of the calories per gram or the energy density, and what this means for food choices, we have divided foods into 4 energy density categories. Remember, the range of energy densities is from 0 to a maximum of 9 calories per gram.

Throughout the book I will give you tips on how to use these categories to guide your food choices. Here are some tips to get you started.

- To decrease calorie intake and feel full on fewer calories, choose foods mostly from Category 1 (very-low-energy-dense foods) and Category 2 (low-energy-dense foods).
- Incorporate foods from Category 1, such as fruits, vegetables, broth-based soups, and nonfat dairy into your diet whenever you can. Have them before meals, with meals, use them in your favorite recipes, and remember that fruits and vegetables make great snacks.

- Add foods from Category 2 such as low-fat meats, grains, and other low-fat dishes to complete your meals.
- Choose foods from Category 3 (medium-energy-dense foods) less frequently and limit your choices and portions from Category 4 (high-energy-dense foods).

Energy Density Categories

Use these four categories of energy density to guide your food choices. I will give you more specific examples of the foods in each category in the charts on pages 22–23.

Category 1	**Very Low Energy Density**	0 to 0.6	Includes nonstarchy fruits and vegetables, nonfat milk, and broth-based soups.
Category 2	**Low Energy Density**	0.6 to 1.5	Includes starchy fruits and vegetables, grains; breakfast cereals with low-fat milk; low-fat meats, beans and legumes, and low-fat mixed dishes such as chili and spaghetti.
Category 3	**Medium Energy Density**	1.5 to 4.0	Includes meats, cheeses, pizza, french fries, salad dressings, bread, pretzels, ice cream, and cake.
Category 4	**High Energy Density**	4.0 to 9.0	Includes crackers, chips, chocolate candies, cookies, nuts, butter, and oils.

ENERGY DENSITY AND THE NUTRITION FACTS LABEL

Energy density is not listed on the Nutrition Facts label, but I am going to give you some tips on how to rapidly assess and compare the energy density of foods. Remember, energy density is measured as calories per gram, and indicates how much energy you'll get from a certain weight of food. If one food has an energy density of 1.0, while another has an energy density of 2.0, you'll get twice as many calories from the same size serving (or weight) of the second food. Similarly, the same size portion of a food with an energy density of 3.0 would provide three times as many calories as the food with an energy density of 1.0. A food with an energy density of 4.0 . . . well, you get the idea of how this works! As you learn to lower the energy density of your favorite foods, you will be able to eat your usual portion, but with fewer calories. For example, if you are having pancakes for breakfast or brunch, two regular pancakes topped with butter and syrup add up to 400 calories or more, but two of Jennifer's Fruit Smothered Whole-Wheat Buttermilk Pancakes (page 62) provide 270 calories, so you save 130 calories.

Reading food labels is an important strategy to help you lower the energy density of your diet. Almost all food packages include a standardized nutrition label. Think of food labels as a tool that can help you make smart food choices. You can quickly find all of the information you need to easily determine the energy density of a food on the label. Let's look at the Nutrition Facts label. I'll use the Nutrition Facts information from a reduced-fat mozzarella cheese stick as an example to help you learn to calculate energy density. The top portion of the label contains all the information you need: calories and weight in grams for a single serving.

Now comes the fun part: To calculate the energy density, divide the calories by the weight: 60 calories divided by 28 grams equals 2.1 calories per gram. Even if you don't have a calculator and aren't good at math in your head, don't worry! You can get a good idea of a food's energy density by simply comparing calories to grams per serving. If the calories are less than the grams, that food has an energy density below 1.0 calorie per gram. If the calories are twice the grams (such as 200 calories in 100 grams), that food has an energy density of 2.0 calories per gram. Use this quick method to compare foods when you're shopping:

Calculating energy density

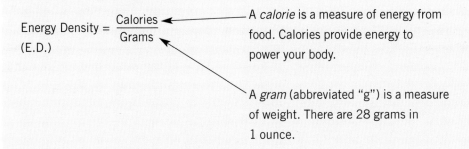

$$\text{Energy Density} = \frac{\text{Calories}}{\text{Grams}}$$
(E.D.)

A *calorie* is a measure of energy from food. Calories provide energy to power your body.

A *gram* (abbreviated "g") is a measure of weight. There are 28 grams in 1 ounce.

Let's look at an example. The Energy Density of a reduced-fat mozzarella stick is 2.1.

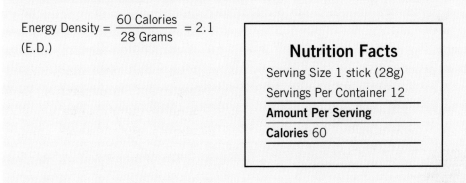

$$\text{Energy Density} = \frac{60 \text{ Calories}}{28 \text{ Grams}} = 2.1$$
(E.D.)

Nutrition Facts

Serving Size 1 stick (28g)

Servings Per Container 12

Amount Per Serving

Calories 60

- **Calories fewer than grams:** Go for it—you can eat satisfying portions.
- **Calories the same or up to twice as many as grams:** Start using portion control.
- **Calories more than twice the grams:** Limit your portions.

You can also use your list of the energy density values for food in the Energy Density Charts (pages 22–23). I have made this list into a simple and easy-to-use shopping guide—copy the charts and take them with you. Within each category, the charts list foods from the lowest energy density to the highest, so it's easy to scan down and compare foods. As you shop, compare foods within each category—the lower the energy density, the more satisfaction you will get per portion. The list gives you

Estimating energy density

No calculators necessary! Here is a quick method for estimating energy density. Simply compare the number of calories to the number of grams in a serving and you will know whether you can eat a satisfying portion or whether you have to exert portion control.

Salsa

The calories (15) are *fewer than* the grams (33).

The energy density is less than 1.

Enjoy satisfying portions!

Nutrition Facts
Serving Size 2 tbsp (33g)
Servings Per Container 14
Amount Per Serving
Calories 15

Refried beans

The calories (123) are *almost the same* as the grams (124).

The energy density is about 1.

Start portion control!

Nutrition Facts
Serving Size ½ cup (124g)
Servings Per Container 4
Amount Per Serving
Calories 123

Tuna canned in oil

The calories (112) are *twice* the grams (56).

The energy density is about 2.

Continue portion control!

Nutrition Facts
Serving Size 2 oz (56g)
Servings Per Container 2.5
Amount Per Serving
Calories 112

Crackers

The calories (140) are *more than twice* the grams (30).

The energy density is greater than 2.

Limit portions!

Nutrition Facts
Serving Size 18 crackers (30g)
Servings Per Container 7
Amount Per Serving
Calories 140

a good overview of foods that you can eat without worrying about portions and those that you need to eat more moderately. The energy density of prepared foods can vary by brand, so check labels. The values in the chart are based on average values. I will give you more tips on how to compare the energy density of foods throughout the book.

Remember though, not *every* food choice you make should be determined by energy density, and we are not going to set an upper limit on the energy density of the foods you should be eating. Some nutritious foods can have a medium or even high energy density, such as nuts and olive oil. These are foods that you will probably want to include in your diet in small amounts. And other high-energy dense foods, like chocolate, are too delicious to give up—have a little at the end of dinner as a treat.

I know you are eager to get started but, before we begin developing your personal eating and weight management plan, you need to learn about beverages, portion size, and calories.

BEVERAGES

What about beverages? If water-rich foods fill you up, won't drinks be even better? The answer is no. Many beverages such as soda and juice satisfy thirst, but not hunger. The calories from drinks consumed before a meal or during a meal add on to the food calories. You are unlikely to eat less just because you are drinking calories. One study in my lab found that calorie intake increased significantly when people drank a beverage containing 150 calories with lunch, compared to when they had a calorie-free beverage.

The good news is that many of you will be able to reduce your intake of calorie-laden drinks without feeling much of a sacrifice. Water is your best choice for quenching thirst, but there are lots of other low-calorie beverages. You can try diet soda or a fruit spritzer made by diluting fruit juice with seltzer. Hot or cold tea is fine, but don't load it up with sugar. Coffee on its own is virtually calorie free, but those coffeehouse mixes of coffee, sugar, and fat, such as lattes, can pack a meal's worth of calories into a single drink.

Calories from alcoholic beverages also add on to food calories. Alcohol is high in energy density with 7 calories per gram, and it is often mixed with sugar-laden liquids such as soda or juice. I am not going to ask you to give up alcohol altogether.

Category 1:
Very Low-Energy-Dense Foods
(0 to 0.6 calories per gram)

Remember, if the number of calories is less than the number of grams: go for it—you can eat satisfying portions.

Food	Energy Density
Chicken broth, fat-free	0.07
Gelatin, fruit-flavored, sugar free	0.07
Cucumber	0.13
Celery	0.16
Chicken broth	0.16
Lettuce	0.18
Tomato	0.21
Asparagus	0.24
Mushrooms	0.27
Broccoli	0.28
Strawberries	0.30
Vegetarian vegetable soup	0.30
Grapefruit	0.30
Fennel	0.31
Watermelon	0.32
Green beans	0.35
Cantaloupe	0.35
Milk, nonfat	0.35
Chicken, rice, and vegetable soup	0.38
Winter squash	0.39
Carrots	0.43
Peach	0.43
Applesauce, unsweetened	0.43
Italian dressing, fat-free	0.47
Orange	0.47
Raspberries	0.48
Yogurt, fruit, fat-free, low-calorie sweetener	0.53
Yogurt, plain, fat-free	0.56
Blueberries	0.56
Apples	0.58
Gelatin, fruit-flavored	0.59
Pears	0.59
Milk, whole (3.3 percent)	0.61

Category 2:
Low-Energy-Dense Foods
(0.6 to 1.5 calories per gram)

These foods make up most of what we eat—you can eat satisfying portions at the low end, but start portion control at the high end.

Food	Energy Density
Tofu	0.61
Instant oatmeal, prepared with water	0.62
Mayonnaise, fat-free	0.62
Yogurt, plain, low-fat	0.63
Cottage cheese, fat-free	0.65
Grapes	0.67
Vegetarian chili	0.67
Beans, black	0.78
Green peas	0.78
Corn on the cob (boiled, drained)	0.86
Orange roughy (broiled)	0.89
Banana	0.92
Beans, baked	0.93
Sour cream, fat-free	0.94
Shrimp, boiled or steamed	1.0
Yogurt, frozen, fat-free	1.0
Yogurt, fruit, low-fat	1.0
Cottage cheese, regular (full fat)	1.0
Sweet potato, baked	1.0
Olives	1.1
Bran flakes with 1 percent milk	1.1
Ketchup	1.1
Potato, baked with skin	1.1
Tuna, canned in water	1.2
Cream, half & half	1.3
Yogurt, frozen, fruit varieties	1.3
Rice, white, long-grain, cooked	1.3
Chili con carne	1.3
Ranch dressing, fat-free	1.4
Pasta, cooked	1.4
Avocado	1.4
Ham, extra lean, 5 percent fat	1.5
Spaghetti with meat sauce	1.5

Category 3:
Medium-Energy-Dense Foods
(1.5 to 4.0 calories per gram)

Watch portion size, especially at the high end of this broad range of foods.

Food	Energy Density
Yogurt, frozen, chocolate or vanilla, soft serve	1.6
Egg, hard boiled	1.6
Turkey breast, roasted, no skin	1.6
Chicken breast, roasted, no skin	1.7
Vegetable burger	1.8
Sirloin steak, lean, broiled	1.9
Tuna, canned in oil	2.0
Bean and cheese burrito	2.0
Egg, fried	2.0
Pumpkin pie	2.1
Margarine, low-calorie	2.1
Bread, whole-wheat	2.5
Preserves, jellies and marmalades	2.5
Ice cream, premium	2.5
Angel food cake	2.6
Mozzarella cheese, part-skim	2.6
Ranch dressing, reduced-fat	2.7
Italian bread, white	2.7
Ground beef, lean, broiled	2.7
Bagel, plain	2.8
Cheese pizza	2.9
Muffin, blueberry	2.9
Raisins	3.0
Potatoes, french fried	3.2
Ravioli, cheese	3.2
Mayonnaise, light	3.3
Doughnut, jelly filled	3.4
Cream cheese, full fat	3.5
Italian dressing, full fat	3.6
Chocolate cake with frosting	3.7
Cheese, Swiss or American	3.8
Hard pretzels	3.9
Tortilla chips, baked	3.9

Category 4:
High-Energy-Dense Foods
(4.0 to 9.0 calories per gram)

You need to manage intake from this category by limiting portions or making substitutions.

Food	Energy Density
Potato chips, baked	3.9
Onion rings, battered and fried	4.1
Frosting, white	4.1
Croissant	4.1
Pie crust	4.1
Doughnut, plain	4.1
Graham crackers	4.2
Granola bar	4.3
Popcorn, caramel	4.3
Cheese, Parmesan	4.6
Chocolate chip cookies, homemade	4.6
Creme-filled chocolate sandwich cookies	4.9
Cheese crackers	5.0
Bacon	5.0
Tortilla chips	5.1
Peanut butter, reduced-fat	5.3
Chips, potato or corn	5.4
Milk chocolate bar	5.4
Peanuts, roasted	5.9
Ranch dressing, full fat	5.9
Peanut butter, creamy	5.9
Pecans, dry roasted	6.6
Mayonnaise, regular, full fat	7.2
Butter	7.2
Margarine, stick	7.2
Oil, vegetable	8.8

Calories in beverages

Beverages can be a source of hidden calories. Often beverages sold in "individual" packages, such as a 16-ounce bottle of soda, contain multiple servings. Think about the beverages you had yesterday . . . how many calories did you drink?

Beverage	Amount	Calories	Energy Density
Water or diet soda	8 ounces	0	0.00
	12 ounces	0	
	16 ounces	0	
Light beer	8 ounces	66	0.28
	12 ounces	99	
	16 ounces	132	
Nonfat milk	8 ounces	86	0.35
	12 ounces	129	
	16 ounces	172	
Beer	8 ounces	97	0.41
	12 ounces	146	
	16 ounces	195	
Cola/soda	8 ounces	101	0.41
	12 ounces	152	
	16 ounces	203	
1 percent milk	8 ounces	102	0.42
	12 ounces	153	
	16 ounces	205	
Orange juice	8 ounces	112	0.45
	12 ounces	167	
	16 ounces	223	
2 percent milk	8 ounces	122	0.50
	12 ounces	183	
	16 ounces	244	
Whole milk	8 ounces	149	0.61
	12 ounces	223	
	16 ounces	298	
Wine	8 ounces	165	0.70
	12 ounces	248	
	16 ounces	330	

Drinking a glass of wine with dinner is okay, but remember that a 4-ounce glass has around 85 calories. You have to budget those calories into your plan.

So, be wise when choosing your drinks. Remind yourself that, for every 12-ounce soda you don't drink, you save 150 calories. If you saved 150 calories every day, that could mean up to a 15 pound weight loss in a year!

MANAGING PORTIONS

How do you decide how much you should eat? If you base your portions on what you are served in restaurants, you are getting many more calories than you need. For example, a typical restaurant tuna-salad sandwich weighs more than 10 ounces and can have 680 or more calories. Health experts define an appropriate portion of this food to be 4 ounces, only 290 calories. So, the restaurant is giving you more than twice as many calories as recommended. You may have noticed that restaurant portions have gradually increased in size in recent years. It's not just happening in restaurants; food manufacturers have also been increasing portion sizes. And portions are growing at home too! Comparisons of cookbooks over the years show that the same recipe serves fewer people now than it did 20 years ago. If you are like most people, you are suffering from portion distortion! Studies in my lab have shown that most people eat more when given bigger portions, and are not even aware that they are doing so.

If you cut calories simply by eating smaller portions of every food, you would feel

How to manage portion distortion

If you choose very-low-energy-dense foods, you will not need to worry about large portions. I want you to eat more of these foods. However, as the energy density of food increases, portion control becomes critical for weight management. Here are some simple strategies to help you to manage portions.

- Recognize that portion sizes have been sneaking up in recent years and that you are likely to be served more calories than you need.
- Learn to read nutrition labels so that you know what the suggested serving size is, and how many calories it contains.

- Use energy density as a guide to the calories in portions. Energy density provides a comparison of the calories in the same size portion of different foods. For more satisfying portions, choose lower-energy-density foods.
- Educate yourself by weighing (using a simple kitchen scale) or measuring (with measuring cups) foods. Figure out how much you are eating and the calories in these portions.
- Don't rely on someone else to dish out the right amount of food.
- Follow the guidelines set by the American Dietetic Association and the American Institute for Cancer Research on how to fill your plate—aim to cover ⅔ or more of your plate with plant-based foods such as fruits, vegetables, whole grains, and beans; and the remaining ⅓ or less with lean animal protein.
- Assess your hunger and fullness while you are eating (page 40) and stop when you are full. It is okay to leave food on the plate.
- Eat slowly and experience flavors and textures. Rather than automatically reaching for seconds, relax for a few minutes to see if you are still hungry.
- If you purchase energy-dense snack foods such as chips or cookies, buy the smallest package or individually wrapped portions.
- If you buy large packages of snacks or staples for economy, transfer the contents into smaller, sealable plastic bags or storage containers.
- When making large batches of foods that can be frozen, portion them out into single-serving freezer/microwave containers and freeze them, so you can reheat a quick portion-controlled meal in minutes.
- If you usually prepare more food than you need, learn to cook less or plan to use extras for lunch or other meals like soups or casseroles. Wrap up extra portions right away to avoid temptation.
- Look for small portions on menus or order an appetizer instead of an entrée.
- Remember that it is okay to take food home when eating out.
- Share a portion—this works especially well with desserts.
- Test whether you are portion savvy on a fun website set up by the National Institutes of Health: http://hin.nhlbi.nih.gov/portion/

hungry and deprived. You might have a hard time sticking to this type of eating plan. This is why learning about low-energy-dense foods is so important. While I want you to manage portions of foods that are high in energy density, I want you to eat *larger* portions of foods that have a *very low* energy density (less than 0.6 calories per gram). Foods like broth-based soups and whole fruits and vegetables will provide you with a satisfying portion of food that has few calories. So, while you're lowering your daily calories by cutting back on high-energy-dense foods, you'll be increasing the volume of your diet with low-energy-dense foods. In this way, you still get to eat your normal weight or volume of food and feel satisfied, not deprived.

I am going to show you how to add plenty of low-energy-dense foods to your diet while reducing portions of high-energy-dense foods. You will learn that it's okay to eat more than one serving of low-energy-dense foods. The foods in Category 1, the very low-energy-dense category—are the ones you should reach for whenever you get the munchies. They are good foods to snack on during the day when you feel hungry, because they provide few calories, but fill you up. Eat a low-energy-dense soup, fruit, or salad (with a low-fat dressing) before a meal to help you feel full, so that you eat less of the main course.

DO YOU HAVE TO COUNT CALORIES?

Calories do count. Calories are just a measure of the heat generated by the foods you eat. Your body, like a furnace, has fuel coming in which is burned to give you energy. To stay the same weight, your body needs to balance the calories going in with those going out. To lose weight, you must eat fewer calories than you burn. To affect your energy balance you can work to change both how much fuel you are taking in and how much you are burning.

Yes, I am building up to telling you again that to lose weight you need to eat less and move more! However, you should keep in mind that even small changes in diet and exercise could have a big impact on your weight and your health over time. Think about it—if you ate just 100 fewer calories a day over a year, you could lose 10 pounds! Of course, it works the other way too. Eating just a little extra each day lets the extra weight sneak on. Each pound of fat contains around 3500 calories. So for each pound you want to lose, you will need to take in 3500 fewer calories than your body is using. Sounds like a lot, but small changes add up quickly.

You are probably asking how you know how many calories you are eating. Many

Easy ways to save calories

Instead of	E.D.	Calories	Substitute	E.D.	Calories	Calorie Savings
Medium bagel (1 bagel)	2.8	195	Whole-wheat toast (1 slice)	2.5	62	**133**
Jelly donut (1 doughnut)	3.4	289	*Blueberry Applesauce Muffin* (page 68) (1 muffin)	1.6	123	**166**
Whole milk (8 ounces)	0.61	150	Nonfat milk (8 ounces)	0.35	86	**64**
Premium ice cream (½ cup)	2.5	270	Fat-free frozen yogurt (½ cup)	1.2	80	**190**
Tuna packed in oil (2 ounces)	2.0	110	Tuna packed in water (2 ounces)	1.2	66	**44**
Roasted chicken wings (3 ounces)	2.9	247	Roasted skinless chicken breast (3 ounces)	1.7	140	**107**
Regular soda (12 ounces)	0.41	152	Diet soda (12 ounces)	0	0	**152**

of you have tried counting calories and have found that it gets tedious quickly. The goal of *Volumetrics* is to get you beyond having to count the calories in every morsel you consume. You need to understand where the calories are, and I will help you with that. When you learn how to choose foods wisely, you will be eating a nutritious balance of foods that will leave you full and satisfied without excess calories. Let's get started. In the next chapter, you will discover your own personal weight management plan.

The principles of *Volumetrics*

What is the ideal weight-loss plan? It is one that satisfies hunger, reduces calories, includes a wide variety of foods, meets nutritional needs, and includes physical activity. It also must be enjoyable and sustainable.

Element	Recommendation	Comments
Energy (Calories)	Reduce usual intake by 500 to 1000 calories a day	This should lead to weight loss of 1 to 2 pounds a week.
Fat	20 to 30 percent of total calories	Choose low-fat or reduced-fat foods with a low energy density.
Carbohydrates	55 percent or more of total calories	To increase satiety emphasize carbohydrates from whole grains, vegetables, and fruits.
Fiber	25 grams a day for women, 38 grams for men	Enjoy lots of whole grains such as fiber-rich breakfast cereals. Fiber helps lower energy density and increases satiety.
Sugars	Choose a diet moderate in sugars	Decrease intake of sugar-based drinks, which add calories with little satiety.
Protein	15 to 35 percent of calories, about 0.4 grams per pound of body weight. You can go up to 0.8 grams per pound if you are very active.	More satiating than carbohydrates or fat. During weight loss, adequate amounts help prevent muscle loss and thus maintain metabolic rate. Choose beans, low-fat fish, and lean meats.
Alcohol	Limit to 1 drink a day for women, 2 for men	Consume with low-energy-dense meals.
Water	Drink about 9 cups of fluids a day for women, 13 for men. This includes water and other beverages.	Replace sugary drinks with water or calorie-free beverages.
Physical activity	Aim for 30 to 60 minutes of modest-intensity physical activity on most days. Include resistance training twice a week.	Many everyday activities can help you reach this goal. Time spent gardening, walking, housekeeping, and using the stairs adds up quickly. Use a step counter!

2 Your Personal Weight Management Plan

I n this chapter, I am going to take you through the basics of weight management and help you develop a personalized plan that fits with your preferences and goals. You are going to start with Week 0. During this week you will establish your baseline, which will determine what you are currently eating and how active you are. You should read through this book and *The Volumetrics Weight-Control Plan* to familiarize yourself with the basic principles of *Volumetrics*. After the baseline week, I will guide you through four weeks of menu planning and goal setting. This will help you to learn about what and how much you should be eating to achieve your goals. You will also be eased into being more active. If you don't feel that you need that much structure, but would rather apply the *Volumetrics* principles in your own way, that is fine, too. Just keep track of your progress—studies show this is critical for successful weight management.

Here is another success story from a reader of *The Volumetrics Weight-Control Plan*:

Dear Dr. Rolls,
I was diagnosed with type II diabetes last February. One of the first things I did was consult a nutritionist. I needed to lose about 70 pounds and I needed help. I remember asking the nutritionist what I can do to stop being hungry all the time. She really did not answer that question. I started experimenting with Volumetrics *before I was even aware that it had a name and that you were the leading proponent of this dietary*

lifestyle. I started eating a big salad as part of dinner every night. Then I began creating meals that filled a soup bowl but were low in calories. Then I found out about your book. As I read it, I realized that I had been practicing what you were preaching without even knowing it. It just makes sense. I now recommend your book to everyone who wants to know my "secret" for losing 70 pounds and there are quite a few who want to know. I would like to see Volumetrics become a household word and will do all I can do in my part of the world to help it happen. Keep up your excellent work.

Heartfelt Thanks,
Pam Cobo

WEEK 0

During this baseline week I am going to show you how to use a chart to keep track of your personal goals. I have started by filling in the chart to give you an example of reasonable goals. In the following pages, I will take you through these goals so you can determine your own personal plan.

Setting achievable goals is an important component of your personal weight management plan. You may fantasize about looking like a model or returning to a younger you, but be realistic. Don't set yourself up for disappointment. True, some people achieve phenomenal weight loss, but many plateau somewhere between losing 5 to 10 percent of their current weight. That amount of weight loss will have brought them many important health benefits: fasting blood sugar levels associated with diabetes will be reduced, blood pressure will have dropped, and the risk factors associated with heart disease will have improved. So think of a loss of 5 to 10 percent of your current weight as a realistic goal. To determine what 5 or 10 percent of your current weight is, follow the instructions in the chart (page 34). When you have calculated your goal weight, add it to your baseline goals chart (page 33). If you find you can lose more than that, you can reset the goal later. Remember to congratulate yourself for any weight loss, and focus on your long-term goals of continuing to eat nutritiously and keep active.

Here is an example of realistic goals.

Week 0 (Baseline)		Goals	
Age:	_35 years_		
Waist size: (page 36)	_42 inches_		
Weight:	_165 pounds_	Goal weight:	_149 pounds_
BMI: (page 35)	_27_	Goal BMI:	_24_
Daily calorie requirement: (page 43)	_2324 calories_	Daily calorie goal:	_1824 calories_
Daily step count: (page 46)	_4,500 steps_	Initial Daily step goal: Long-term step goal:	_6,500 steps_ _10,000 steps_

Use this goals chart for your own goals.

Week 0 (Baseline)		Goals	
Age:	_51_		
Waist size:			
Weight:	_157 160_	Goal weight:	_145_
BMI:	_26 26_	Goal BMI:	_24_
Daily calorie requirement:	_2000_	Daily calorie goal:	_1600_
Daily step count:	_6000_	Initial Daily step goal: Long-term step goal:	_10000_

Calculate your weight loss goal

EXAMPLE

If you weigh 165 pounds, 10% of your body weight is 16 pounds

____165____ pounds X 0.10 = ____16____ pounds
(current body weight)   (10% of your body weight)

Your goal weight would be 149 pounds.

____165____ pounds – ____16____ pounds = ____149____ pounds
(current body weight)   (10% of your body weight)

NOW IT IS YOUR TURN

10% of your body weight: (for a 5% weight loss substitute 0.05 for 0.10)

____157____ pounds X 0.10 = ____15____ pounds
(current body weight)   (10% of your body weight)

Your goal weight.

____157____ pounds – ____15____ pounds = ____142____ pounds
(current body weight)   (10% of your body weight)

Now, let's set a few more goals related to your body size. Just as you should know your cholesterol levels and your blood pressure, you should be aware of your body-mass index (BMI) and your waist measurement. Both of these numbers can give you an idea of whether you are overweight. Your BMI is a ratio that indicates whether your weight is appropriate for your height. It reflects body fat in most adults, the exception being very fit people who weigh more because they are muscular. You can look up your BMI on the chart (page 35) using your height and current weight. To determine your goal BMI, use your goal weight you just calculated. If you are 5 feet and 6 inches tall, and your current weight is 165, your BMI is 27. With a goal weight of 149 pounds, the goal BMI would be 24.

Use this chart to determine your BMI by finding the intersection of your weight and your height.

Weight / Height	100	105	110	115	120	125	130	135	140	145	150	155	160	165	170	175	180	185	190	195	200	205	210	215	220	225	230	235	240	245	250
5'0"	20	21	21	22	23	24	25	26	27	28	29	30	31	32	33	34	35	36	37	38	39	40	41	42	43	44	45	46	47	48	49
5'1"	19	20	21	22	23	24	25	26	26	27	28	29	30	31	32	33	34	35	36	37	38	39	40	41	42	43	43	44	45	46	47
5'2"	18	19	20	21	22	23	24	25	26	27	27	28	29	30	31	32	33	34	35	36	37	37	38	39	40	41	42	43	44	45	46
5'3"	18	19	19	20	21	22	23	24	25	26	27	27	28	29	30	31	32	33	34	35	35	36	37	38	39	40	41	42	43	43	44
5'4"	17	18	19	20	21	21	22	23	24	25	26	27	27	28	29	30	31	32	33	33	34	35	36	37	38	39	39	40	41	42	43
5'5"	17	17	18	19	20	21	22	22	23	24	25	26	27	27	28	29	30	31	32	32	33	34	35	36	37	37	38	39	40	41	42
5'6"	16	17	18	19	19	20	21	22	23	23	24	25	26	27	27	28	29	30	31	31	32	33	34	35	35	36	37	38	39	39	40
5'7"	16	16	17	18	19	20	20	21	22	23	23	24	25	26	27	27	28	29	30	30	31	32	33	34	34	35	36	37	38	38	39
5'8"	15	16	17	17	18	19	20	20	21	22	23	24	24	25	26	27	27	28	29	30	30	31	32	33	33	34	35	36	36	37	38
5'9"	15	15	16	17	18	18	19	20	21	21	22	23	24	24	25	26	27	27	28	29	30	30	31	32	32	33	34	35	35	36	37
5'10"	14	15	16	17	17	18	19	19	20	21	22	22	23	24	24	25	26	27	27	28	29	29	30	31	32	32	33	34	34	35	36
5'11"	14	15	15	16	17	17	18	19	20	20	21	22	22	23	24	24	25	26	27	27	28	29	29	30	31	31	32	33	34	34	35
6'0"	14	14	15	16	16	17	18	18	19	20	20	21	22	22	23	24	24	25	26	27	27	28	29	29	30	31	31	32	33	33	34
6'1"	13	14	15	15	16	16	17	18	18	19	20	20	21	22	22	23	24	24	25	26	26	27	28	28	29	30	30	31	32	32	33
6'2"	13	13	14	15	15	16	17	17	18	19	19	20	21	21	22	22	23	24	24	25	26	26	27	28	28	29	30	30	31	31	32
6'3"	12	13	14	14	15	16	16	17	17	18	19	19	20	21	21	22	22	23	24	24	25	26	26	27	27	28	29	29	30	31	31
6'4"	12	13	13	14	15	15	16	16	17	18	18	19	19	20	21	21	22	23	23	24	24	25	26	26	27	27	28	29	29	30	30

Underweight	Normal weight	Overweight	Obese

Here's how to interpret your BMI.

- **BMI under 18.5.** You are underweight. You should not consider dieting; it could endanger your health.
- **BMI of 18.5 to 24.9.** You are at a healthy weight. Your goals should include maintaining your weight by eating nutritiously and being active.
- **BMI of 25 to 29.9.** You are overweight. At this level the risk to your health is modest, but you should strive to not gain any more weight. Health risks rise with a BMI over 27.
- **BMI of 30 to 34.9.** You are obese. Your health risks are increased so you need to take action now to improve your health. Remember that even small decreases in your BMI can be beneficial.
- **BMI over 35.** At this level of obesity you should talk to your physician about weight loss.

At any BMI, you are at increased risk of heart disease and diabetes if you carry your weight around your middle. This is an apple shape, as opposed to a pear, which carries weight around the hips and thighs. Specifically, a waist size of over 35 inches in women and 40 inches in men is associated with increased risk. To measure your waist size, wrap a tape measure around your middle at the top of your hipbones. It should feel snug, but shouldn't push your skin in. Take the measurement after you exhale. This may not be your natural waist or the smallest part of your waist. If you are having trouble, ask a friend to help. People vary in how their body shape changes with weight loss. Any decrease in your waist size will be beneficial. Tracking changes in your waist measurement can help keep you motivated.

CALCULATING YOUR DAILY CALORIE NEEDS

To get started with this plan you need to have an idea of what you are currently eating. Successful weight management programs often start with clients keeping careful records of everything they are eating. Such records are particularly helpful in finding areas where your eating habits can improve. They challenge you to ask yourself where you can easily make changes and where you would have difficulty. You should copy the Food Diary form (page 38) and use it to examine what you are eating

Sample *Volumetrics* food diary

Date <u>Aug 17</u>

Time	Food	Amount	E. D. Category	Improvement Strategies
7:30	Orange juice	1 cup	1	Substitute a whole orange.
7:30	Coffee with cream	1 cup	1	Use milk.
7:30	English muffin with butter	2	3	Substitute fiber-rich breakfast cereal with low-fat milk.
10:30	Chocolate cream-filled sandwich cookies	6	4	Pack and snack on an apple.
12:30	Baked potato with butter and cheese sauce	1	3	Top the potato with steamed broccoli and salsa.
12:30	Ham and cheese sandwich	1	3	Use whole-wheat bread. Add more vegetables. Use mustard or reduced-fat mayo.
3:30	Potato chips	1 small bag	4	Pack and snack on low-fat yogurt or a reduced-fat cheese stick.
6:00	Thick-crust pizza with extra meat and cheese	3 slices	3	Start dinner with a low-energy-dense soup and salad. Eat fewer slices of pizza. Order thin-crust pizza with extra veggies.
8:00	Milk shake	1 cup	2	Have a fresh fruit smoothie.

Volumetrics food diary

Date _____

A blank food diary for you to copy and use to keep track of what you are eating.

Time	Food	Amount	E. D. Category	Improvement Strategies

each day during the baseline week. I've filled in a sample Food Diary form (page 37) as a guide.

I am asking you to fill in the energy density categories of the foods you are eating. This will help you to learn about the energy density of different foods and will also show you where you can make changes that will lower the energy density of your diet. In Chapter 1, you learned how to calculate energy density values using food labels (page 19). You can also use the shopping charts in Chapter 1 (pages 22–23) and the modular lists in Chapter 15 (pages 273–92) to find energy density values.

Now that you have seven days of food records, let's consider what you should look for when reviewing them.

- Are most of your food choices from Categories 1 and 2? It's okay to eat foods from Categories 3 and 4 but you should monitor your portions.
- Are you eating foods in energy density Categories 3 and 4 that you can give up or eat less often? Or can you reduce the energy density of some foods by changing the preparation method; for example, have grilled instead of fried fish. Look for other places where you can cut the fat.
- Did you eat a good variety of foods? Variety is key for optimal nutrition in that it helps ensure you get a balance of nutrients. Your diet should include plenty of fruits and vegetables, whole grains, low-fat dairy products, and varied sources of protein such as legumes, fish, and *lean* meat.
- Where can you add more vegetables and fruits? What about your snacks? Can you take an apple to work to help you resist the vending machines?
- Are you drinking too many caloric beverages such as soda, fruit juice, or alcoholic beverages? These add on to your food calories. Cutting calories from beverages is an easy change to make since there are so many tasty low-calorie or even zero-calorie beverages.
- Is your eating distributed across the day? You should aim for the standard three meals with two nutritious snacks. This is the most typical eating pattern and it will help to keep your hunger under control.
- Do you skip meals? Going too long without eating can lead to loss of control over how much you eat later.

Remember as you evaluate your food records that you are looking for ways to make improvements you can sustain. During the next 4 weeks, you will use these

Get in touch with feelings of hunger and satiety

Have you lost touch with what your body is trying to tell you about when to eat and how much to eat? If so, I am going to show you how to start listening again. You should start with slowing down at each meal and paying attention. It is appropriate to feel hungry before each meal. Most people describe hunger as stomach growls and stomach aches. You should not get so hungry that you feel dizzy and light-headed, or that you lose control of your eating. While you are eating, hunger should decline and you should feel pleasantly, but not overly, full. If you don't recognize or experience this cycle of hunger and fullness, try the following:

- For two days this week, ask yourself before each meal, "Am I hungry?"
- Use the scale below to rate your hunger on a scale of 1 to 10, 1 being painfully ravenous and 10 being so full you couldn't eat another bite.

Am I hungry?
Ravenous   1   2   3   4   5   6   7   8   9   10   Completely full

- As you eat, periodically pause and ask yourself, "Am I still hungry?"
- If your rating has reached 5, it may be time to stop eating. Ratings in the middle of the scale should indicate that you are no longer hungry nor are you overly full—you should be comfortable.
- If you are starting to feel full and satisfied, stop eating for 15 minutes, allowing yourself time to recognize your body's satiety signals.
- If you still feel hungry, continue eating while monitoring your feelings of hunger and fullness.
- If you are really out of touch with hunger and satiety, try this routine. Eat breakfast, lunch, and dinner on a regular schedule for several days and don't snack. You should feel hungry before meals and satiated after meals. Use the rating scale before each meal and pay attention to how you feel. Remember these feelings and use them to guide your future eating.

baseline records to set goals to improve your eating habits. While you are following the four-week menu plan you will be exploring new foods and learning about techniques to modify foods.

Thus far, I have had you focus on the types of foods you eat, but you should also think about your eating behavior. I want you to pay attention to what you are eating and savor each bite—mindless eating means extra calories. To experience appropriate satiety, you need to pay attention to what you are eating, and to learn to eat appropriate amounts to satisfy hunger. Your personal goals should include strategies to improve both what you eat and how you are eating. This baseline period is a good time to see if you are in touch with hunger and satiety. I show you how on page 40.

You may be wondering why I have not suggested that you try to calculate your daily calorie intake from the records. You can certainly do that—there are computer programs that can help—but, even with help from technology, the calculations can be time consuming. While your baseline calorie intake can be calculated from your diet records, you can get a good idea of how many calories you should eat each day by using the daily energy requirements worksheet based on recommendations from the Institute of Medicine (page 43). You should use a step counter to measure your activity level before determining your daily energy requirements (page 46). The number of steps is based on a walking speed of about 3 miles per hour. After you calculate your daily calorie needs, record it on page 33.

I want you to lose weight at a slow and steady rate of 1 to 2 pounds per week. I know you want to get to your goal weight by yesterday, but remember that slow and steady weight loss is more likely to be maintained than rapid weight loss. To lose a pound a week, you need to shave 500 calories from your calculated daily intake— 2 pounds requires 1000 calories less per day. Subtract 500 to 1000 calories from your daily calorie requirements to determine your daily calorie goal. Since the formula can only provide an estimate of your calorie needs, you need to monitor your weight loss and adjust your calorie level down if the loss is too little and up if it is too fast. The good news is that as you learn to eat more low-energy-dense foods you will find that you will worry less about monitoring calories.

Sample daily energy requirements worksheet for women

Determine your daily activity level

Sedentary: little walking, stair climbing, gardening or other activity
Low active: 30 to 90 minutes a day brisk activity (~3,600 to 10,800 steps)
Active: 1½ to 3½ hours a day brisk activity (~10,800 to 25,000 steps)
Very active: 3½ or more hours a day brisk activity (~25,000 steps)

1. If your activity level is:

   Sedentary, enter 1.00   _____1.14_____   (A)
   Low active, enter 1.14   (activity level)
   Active, enter 1.27
   Very active, enter 1.45

   > If you spend 45 minutes a day walking briskly, you have a low activity level and would enter a 1.14

2. Multiply your height   _____1107_____   (B)
   (inches) by 16.78   (height x 16.78)

   > If you are 5 foot 6 inches tall, your height in inches is 66.
   > 66 x 16.78 = 1107

3. Multiply your weight   _____817_____   (C)
   (pounds) by 4.95   (weight x 4.95)

   > 165 pounds x 4.95 = 817

   > 35 years x 7.31 = 256

4. Multiply your age   _____256_____   (D)
   (years) by 7.31   (age x 7.31)

   > 1107 + 817 = 1924

5. Add line B and line C   _____1924_____   (E)
   (B + C)

   > 1.14 x 1924 = 2193

   > 387 − 256 = 131

6. Multiply line A by line E   _____2193_____   (F)
   (A x E)

   > 131 + 2193 = 2324
   > Your daily energy needs are 2324 calories. To lose a pound a week, consume 500 calories less, which is 1824 calories.

7. Subtract line D from 387   _____131_____   (G)
   (387 − D)

8. Add line G and line F   2324 calories
   (G + F)

Daily energy requirements worksheet

Determine your daily activity level

Sedentary: little walking, stair climbing, gardening or other activity
Low active: 30 to 90 minutes a day brisk activity (~3,600 to 10,800 steps)
Active: 1½ to 3½ hours a day brisk activity (~10,800 to 25,000 steps)
Very active: 3½ or more hours a day brisk activity (~25,000 steps)

WOMEN

1. If your activity level is:
   Sedentary, enter 1.00 _____ (A)
   Low active, enter 1.14 (activity level)
   Active, enter 1.27
   Very active, enter 1.45
2. Multiply your height _____ (B)
   (inches) by 16.78   (height x 16.78)
3. Multiply your weight _____ (C)
   (pounds) by 4.95   (weight x 4.95)
4. Multiply your age _____ (D)
   (years) by 7.31   (age x 7.31)
5. Add line B and line C _____ (E)
   (B + C)
6. Multiply line A by _____ (F)
   line E   (A x E)
7. Subtract line D _____ (G)
   from 387   (387 – D)
8. Add line G and line F _____
   (G + F)

MEN

1. If your activity level is:
   Sedentary, enter 1.00 _____ (A)
   Low active, enter 1.12 (activity level)
   Active, enter 1.27
   Very active, enter 1.54
2. Multiply your height _____ (B)
   (inches) by 12.8   (height x 12.8)
3. Multiply your weight _____ (C)
   (pounds) by 6.46   (weight x 6.46)
4. Multiply your age _____ (D)
   (years) by 9.72   (age x 9.72)
5. Add line B and _____ (E)
   line C   (B + C)
6. Multiply line A _____ (F)
   by line E   (A x E)
7. Subtract line D _____ (G)
   from 864   (864 – D)
8. Add line G and line F _____
   (G + F)

This is the estimated number of calories you need to maintain your current weight

ESTABLISHING GOALS FOR PHYSICAL ACTIVITY

Increasing physical activity is an important part of your weight management program. Reducing calories to lose weight causes you to lose not just body fat but also lean body mass, primarily muscle. Yet muscle is your metabolic secret weapon. Muscle is very active tissue; even at rest, a pound of muscle burns more calories than a pound of body fat. Muscle also smoothes and firms your body shape, so it makes sense to conserve your lean body mass while losing weight. Consider the benefits of exercise.

- Increasing physical activity slows the loss of lean body mass during weight loss.
- You not only burn calories during exercise, but also keep burning them at a higher rate for several hours after you exercise.
- Exercise builds muscle. Resistance or weight training is particularly effective at building muscle, but any aerobic activity that works the long muscles of the legs and arms (walking, jogging, swimming, cross-country skiing) helps too.
- Physical activity also helps people make a commitment to a healthier lifestyle.

Regular physical activity is one of the most reliable ways to boost your mood, lower anxiety, curb depression, improve sleep, and enhance your self-esteem. It makes you feel good, and that's been shown to help in sticking with a weight-loss program. Sustained physical activity is helpful in the prevention of weight regain. In addition, even moderate physical activity helps to reduce the risk of cardiovascular disease and diabetes beyond what weight reduction alone can do.

The most important strategy for you to ensure you fit activity into your day is to find what you enjoy. Keeping fit and healthy is not meant to be drudgery—it has to be fun. So move in any way that you like—here I'm going to show you how simply walking more can be of benefit. While I am focusing on walking, if that is not your preferred activity, that is okay. Just keep track of your activities and set goals to maintain or increase them.

Stepping Up Your Activity

Every day, you take steps. You may walk around a store, to your car, or to the corner. You don't need a gym, a track, or a park to take steps—you can do it almost anywhere. If you add a few steps to your regular routine, throughout your day, you're treating your body to more exercise.

I encourage you to buy and wear a pedometer, a simple device that you can put on your waistband to count the number of steps you take. You can find one in most sporting goods stores. Don't buy one of the cheapest ones—they tend to be inaccurate. Your best choice is one that is simple to use—don't go for lots of extras like calorie counting. The counter gives you a measure of your daily activity, and many people have found it helps motivate them to move more. Increasing physical activity through adding steps is a fun, easy way to take care of your body and improve the quality of your life. You'll be surprised by how many steps you already take in a day—it's probably more than you think! Use your step counter to keep track of your average daily steps. Then, once you're ready to add steps throughout your day, you can watch your step numbers grow!

Increasing your steps doesn't take a large time commitment. Just keep doing what you're doing, and log a few more steps every day with your step counter. If you want to take your extra steps all at one time, you can. Otherwise, it's easy to add a few steps here and there. Several shorter periods of walking are as beneficial to your overall health as a longer, sustained walk.

Fun step facts

- 1 mile = 2,000 to 2,500 steps
- 10,000 steps = 4 to 5 miles
- 1 city block is about 200 steps
- Most people walk about 1,200 steps in 10 minutes

When you start, you should determine your baseline, which is the number of steps you usually walk each day. To establish your baseline, wear your step counter for one full week. There's no need to change your regular routine this week.

- **At the beginning of each day:** Reset your step counter by pressing the reset button. Remember to keep your routine the same for now.
- **At the end of each day:** Record the number of steps displayed on your step counter.
- **At the end of seven days:** Add up your total steps over the week and divide by seven. Now, you have your baseline number, and you are ready to set your personal goal.

Use this chart to track how many steps you take each day

	Week 0 Steps
Monday	Number of steps:
Tuesday	Number of steps:
Wednesday	Number of steps:
Thursday	Number of steps:
Friday	Number of steps:
Saturday	Number of steps:
Sunday	Number of steps:
	Total steps over the week =
	Average steps (sum divided by 7) =
	Steps goal (average steps + 2000) =

To set your goal, take your baseline number and simply add 2000 steps to it. For example, if your baseline number is 4500 steps per day, use 6500 as your step goal. Adding 2000 steps may sound like a lot, but it should only take 15 to 20 minutes over the course of your day. At the start of each week, increase your goal number of steps until you reach 10,000 steps per day. This is the minimum recommended number of steps per day. Don't be frustrated if you have trouble reaching 2000 more steps each week. Instead change your goal to 1000 more steps. Even with this goal, most people find they can reach 10,000 steps per day within a few weeks of starting the program.

You may find it fun to join others who are increasing their steps. There is a national movement—America on the Move (www.americaonthemove.org)—that is helping people all over the country to be physically active. Here are more ideas to help you increase your daily steps and meet your personal step goal.

How to increase your steps

At Home
- Walk your dog, or offer to walk your neighbor's dog.
- Walk to your friend's house instead of calling.
- If you make a telephone call, walk while you talk.
- Start a walking club with your neighbors or friends.
- Turn off the television and do something active with your family.
- Plan walks into your day, for example, with a friend at the beginning of the day, and with your family at the end of the day.
- Plan active weekends (longer walks, scenic hikes, playing in the park).

Around Town
- Park farther away in store parking lots.
- Walk, don't drive, for trips under one mile.
- Walk at the airport while waiting for your plane, and bypass the moving walkways.
- Avoid the drive through of a restaurant, pharmacy, or bank. Instead, walk inside.
- Plan active vacations.

At Work

- Get off the bus earlier and walk farther to work.
- Park away from the entrance to your building.
- Host walking meetings, or start a walking club with your coworkers.
- Walk to a restroom, water fountain, or copy machine on a different floor.
- Walk during your lunch break.
- Walk to a colleague's office rather than calling or sending e-mail.
- At least every 30 minutes, get up and take a walking break from your desk.
- Take the stairs rather than the elevator or the escalator.
- Try to take half of your goal steps by noon.

BEHAVIORAL CHALLENGES

You are now ready to get started. Remember that this is not a quick-fix diet plan. I want you to learn how to establish habits that are both healthy and sustainable. Here are some tips on how to achieve this:

Set the right goals—focus on diet and exercise changes that will lead to permanent weight loss. Effective goals follow.

- **Specific:** "I will exercise more" is a fine goal, but not specific enough. Make goals that are specific and measurable, such as "I will walk for 20 minutes, 3 days per week," or "I will try one new vegetable this week."
- **Realistic:** Often when starting a new program, people are very motivated and set overly ambitious goals. When they realize they are unable to meet those goals, they become discouraged and give up on their program. Don't set yourself up for failure. Instead, set realistic small goals that will help you achieve your long-range goals. For example, setting a goal of walking 5 miles everyday is specific and measurable, but is it achievable if you're just starting your walking program, or if you have a very busy schedule? Start with more realistic and attainable goals and work up from there.
- **Forgiving:** If you find that you have made a less-than-ideal food choice or are unable to achieve all of your weekly exercise goals, don't let that lead to self-

defeating thoughts and feelings. Try to handle it in a more constructive way. For example, if you have a doughnut on the way to work, you might think that you've really blown it and that you might as well eat whatever you want that day. Instead of giving up for the day, decide to make healthier choices at lunch and dinner so that you still are successful for the day. If you miss a day of walking because of a busy schedule or bad weather, forgive yourself and add small amounts of other activities into your day, such as taking the stairs instead of the elevator.

Learn *cue control*. This involves learning which social or environmental cues encourage undesired eating, and then taking steps to change those cues. For example, you may learn that you're more likely to overeat when watching television, when treats are on display by the office coffee pot, or when around a certain friend. Here are some ways to change stimulus or cue situations.

- **Separate the association of eating from specific cues:** For example, don't eat while watching television. Decide to eat only in certain rooms of the house, such as the kitchen or dining room.
- **Avoid or eliminate the cue:** If you find certain foods such as chocolate, cookies, cheese, or chips are too easy to overeat, keep them out of the house entirely, and eat them only on special occasions. If there are treats near the office coffee pot, leave the coffee room immediately after pouring coffee. Bring a healthy Volumetrics snack with you to eat instead.

WEEKS 1 TO 4

I know you are anxious to get started, but you will be glad that you charted your baseline behavior so you can look back and congratulate yourself on your achievements. The next step is to turn to Chapter 15 where you will find a 4-week menu plan that you can adjust to different calorie levels (pages 269–272). By following this plan, you will eliminate the need to count calories, and you will learn about appropriate food choices and how much you should be eating. This is meant to guide your food choices over the next 3 weeks. You can follow the plan exactly or, since each meal is set to a certain calorie level, you can mix and match meals from different days. I'm sure you will find some meals that you enjoy so much you will want to have them more frequently. During Week 4, you will create your own plan based on the foods you have found that fit into your lifestyle.

My hope is that you won't have to worry about counting calories when you are familiar with the *Volumetrics* way of eating. In my lab, we conducted a weight-loss trial in which we taught people about how to reduce the energy density of their diet without any calorie counting. The participants achieved weight loss that was equal to the best results seen in other weight-loss studies. They did this by making the right food choices in appropriate portions, by moving more, and by setting manageable personal goals. You can do this too!

Here is what I want you to do while following the menu plan:

- Use the daily self-monitoring form What I Ate to keep track of what you are eating. I give you an example of how simple this can be. Copy the form on page 53 for your own use. This includes keeping a simple list of foods you have eaten to make sure you are aware of what you are eating. As I mentioned before, keeping track of what you are eating is associated with successful weight management. I've been keeping brief lists of what I eat for years. Thinking about the foods you eat will help you to make smart choices in the future. Since you are following the menu plan, you don't need to worry about calories and energy density.

Example of daily self-monitoring form: What I ate.

	BREAKFAST	SNACK	LUNCH	SNACK	DINNER	SNACK	BEVERAGES
Monday	• cereal with milk	• grapes	• buffalo-chicken wrap • insalata mista • apple	• mozzarella stick	• salad • red beans and rice • wheat roll	• pear	• milk • water • diet cola

- Keep track of whether or not your meals were full of foods with a low energy density and if your eating was guided by hunger and satiety on the Self-monitoring form: How am I doing? (page 54). Record whether you met your goals or whether you could improve. Concentrate on when and where you are eating. Focus on regular eating times, and rate your hunger as you eat. Eat sitting at a table rather than in front of the TV. Check out the example of this form to see how easy this can be.

Example of daily self-monitoring form: How am I doing?

WEIGHT: 162 POUNDS

	Meals: were they full of low ED foods?	Hunger and satiety guided your eating.	Daily steps	Favorite volumetric meals & snacks	Daily personal goal
Monday	☒ Yes ☐ Mostly ☐ Improve	☐ Yes ☒ Mostly ☐ Improve	8,028	• Santa Fe Steak Salad • hummus	Pack my lunch and snacks.

- Record your daily steps. Each day think of new ways to sneak in a few more steps.
- Make sure to note the foods that you especially like on the self-monitoring form: How am I doing? (page 54). This will be very useful for future meal and snack planning. When you are using the modular list to select snacks, carefully choose those that will help you resist high-calorie options. Make a note of what you liked and what kept you from getting too hungry before the next meal.
- Write down a personal goal each day. Make sure it is realistic. For example, resolve that you will take the stairs instead of the elevator at least once a day. Build on the goals from previous days. Each week have a goal of trying one new fruit and one new vegetable.
- You should keep track of your weight. An example is filled in on page 52. Copy the blank chart (page 55) and keep it by your scale. I know some programs say you should not weigh yourself too often, and certainly not more than once a week. But studies show that frequent self-monitoring, not only of intake and activity, but also of weight are associated with success. A basic guide is that you

should weigh yourself, and record that weight at least once a week. You should not weigh yourself more than once a day—the numbers will simply reflect what you just ate or your fluid balance. So, decide how often you want to weigh yourself, realizing that fluctuations of several pounds from day to day are normal and do not necessarily reflect how well you are doing on the plan. Be sure to weigh yourself at the same time each day, preferably without clothes. Look for a general downward trend of 1 to 2 pounds per week with some fluctuations.

- Weight loss often slows or even stops after the first several weeks. Don't be discouraged if this happens. You may need to lower your calorie intake or increase your activity. Recognize that such plateaus are normal, and focus on not regaining lost weight.

Example of how to plot your weight loss success!

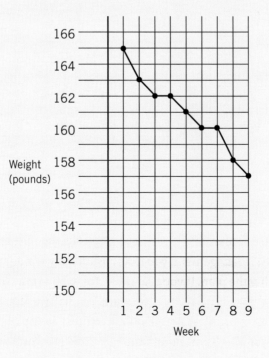

Daily self-monitoring form: What I ate.

	Breakfast	Snack	Lunch	Snack	Dinner	Snack	Beverages
Monday							
Tuesday							
Wednesday							
Thursday							
Friday							
Saturday							
Sunday							

AFTER WEEK 4

If you have followed the menu plan, and if you have increased your activity level and set realistic goals for weight management, you now have the knowledge to do it on your own, without following the plan. If you find it helpful to have the structure, terrific—keep going with the menu plan. I am sure that you will want to tinker with it to emphasize the foods that you liked and that fit your lifestyle. My hope is that while following the plan, you will have learned the types and amounts of foods that will help you manage your weight.

Daily self-monitoring form: How am I doing?

Weight: _____

	Meals: Were they full of low ED foods?	Hunger and satiety guided your eating.	Daily steps	Favorite volumetric meals & snacks	Daily personal goal
Monday	☐ Yes ☐ Mostly ☐ Improve	☐ Yes ☐ Mostly ☐ Improve			
Tuesday	☐ Yes ☐ Mostly ☐ Improve	☐ Yes ☐ Mostly ☐ Improve			
Wednesday	☐ Yes ☐ Mostly ☐ Improve	☐ Yes ☐ Mostly ☐ Improve			
Thursday	☐ Yes ☐ Mostly ☐ Improve	☐ Yes ☐ Mostly ☐ Improve			
Friday	☐ Yes ☐ Mostly ☐ Improve	☐ Yes ☐ Mostly ☐ Improve			
Saturday	☐ Yes ☐ Mostly ☐ Improve	☐ Yes ☐ Mostly ☐ Improve			
Sunday	☐ Yes ☐ Mostly ☐ Improve	☐ Yes ☐ Mostly ☐ Improve			

Plot your weight loss success!

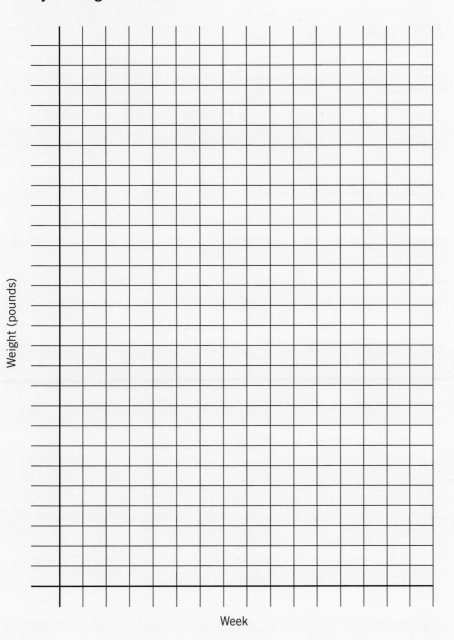

Weight (pounds)

Week

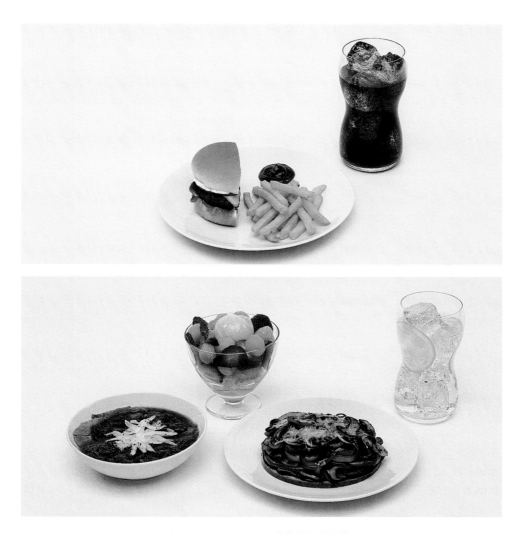

How can you take your favorite meal and make it Volumetric? Both of the lunches pictured above have 500 calories. Which would be more satisfying—half a hamburger, a few fries, and a soda or an Open-Faced Roast Beef Sandwich (page 118), Rustic Tomato Soup (page 101), Four Fruit Compote (page 249), and sparkling water?

Here are a few tips to remind you of what you should be doing to continue to manage your weight.

- If you choose foods low in energy density, you will be eating satisfying portions while reducing your calorie intake. Choose most of your foods from Categories 1 and 2 and you will not have to worry about counting calories.
- Follow the tips throughout this book so that you will make nutritious choices that will enhance satiety.
- Continue to monitor what you are eating, your activity, and goals. You can cut down on the amount of detail in your food diary and simply use it to remind yourself of what you are eating.
- Continue to chart your weight. Remember you are aiming to lose a pound per week.
- Celebrate your success and accept that some setbacks are inevitable. Look beyond your short-term goals to a long-term goal of eating a healthy diet and keeping active.

At some point, you will decide that you no longer wish to continue losing weight. This could be because you reached your goal, or it could be that you are happy with what you have achieved. Many people find losing weight to be easier than keeping it off. Psychologically, it is easier to congratulate yourself when the numbers on the scale keep going down than it is to celebrate the same weight week after week. You need to change that way of thinking. Avoiding weight gain or regain is one of the most important and healthy achievements in weight management. If you have followed *The Volumetrics Eating Plan* so far, you should have a pretty good idea of what is sustainable. I have encouraged you to keep track of favorite foods and menus and to find ways to sneak activity into your day. You need to continue with these favorites and keep trying to find new healthy foods and different activities that you really like.

Self-monitoring has been shown to be more important than ever during maintenance. Continue to use the simplified food record and weight charts to keep track of how you are doing. Remember that successful maintenance is not only easier, but much more likely if you stay physically active. Recent research shows that those who consistently adhere to their eating and activity plan are the most successful at keeping the weight off. The longer you maintain your weight loss, the better the chances that you will achieve long-term success.

3 Breakfast

Mom was right—you shouldn't even *think* about skipping breakfast! Having a strategy to ensure that you eat breakfast every morning is an important part of weight management. Plan ahead and lay out your breakfast the night before, or wake up just a few minutes earlier. By sitting down to breakfast, you can easily increase your intake of vitamins, minerals, and fiber. Eating whole-grains at breakfast is associated with a number of health benefits, such as reduced risk of diabetes and heart disease. Eating breakfast also helps to restore blood glucose levels that fall overnight, leaving you more energized and alert. If you are trying to lose weight, you may think skipping breakfast is an easy way to save some calories. Numerous studies have shown this logic to be wrong. Instead, research has shown that eating breakfast is an important strategy for weight management. Consider the following.

- People who skip breakfast end up eating more later in the day when they are surrounded by energy-dense convenience foods.
- Regular breakfast eaters have a lower body weight than those who skip breakfast.
- Women on a weight-loss diet who ate breakfast lost more weight in three months than those who skipped breakfast.
- The National Weight Control Registry, which tracks several thousand men and women who have successfully maintained a weight loss of at least 30 pounds for a year, finds that 78 percent of them eat breakfast every day.

If all of this evidence is not enough to convince you of the importance of eating breakfast, consider the example you set for your children. Skipping breakfast is associated with overweight in children—and this habit is likely to carry on into adulthood. Children who eat breakfast perform better in school. They are more creative, have better language skills, and have better problem-solving abilities.

Research not only shows the benefits of eating breakfast, it also points to the best choices for weight management. These choices fit right in with the principles of Volumetrics.

Cereals: Choose high-fiber, whole-grain cereals. High-fiber cereals have been shown to enhance satiety and to reduce calorie intake at lunch. Look for cereals that have at least 3 grams of fiber per serving. Go for cereals with lower sugar content, and add as little sugar as you can to still enjoy the meal. It can be tricky to estimate appropriate portions of cereals. Flaky or puffed cereals fill the bowl with fewer calories than those that pack down, such as granola. If you fill your bowl to the same level, granola will give you three times as many calories as cornflakes! Use the recommended serving size on the box as a guide for how much cereal to eat in relation to your calorie goals. A bowl of cereal with low-fat milk is a better choice than cereal bars, which are high in energy density.

Calcium: Add low-fat milk or yogurt to lower the energy density of breakfast and increase calcium intake. In addition to helping you have healthy bones, a number of studies have shown that adequate calcium intake (1000 to 1300 mg per day depending on your age) is an important component of a successful weight management plan. It appears that calcium, particularly from dairy products, may help you burn fat. Remember, for weight management, the key is to eat adequate amounts of calcium. Eating more will not increase the benefit. Make sure when choosing dairy products to look for those low in fat. The fat and calories in milk add up quickly, so you should gradually shift to milk with a lower percent fat—it can take several months to prefer drinking it to the milk you drank previously. Gradually continue to change the type of milk you drink until you reach nonfat milk. Choosing nonfat milk over whole milk saves you 64 calories per 8-ounce glass.

Fruit: Eating more fruit at breakfast helps to lower the energy density, and adds fiber and nutrients. Remember whole fruit provides more fiber than juice. Start your meal with a juicy orange or half a grapefruit. You can also add berries or melon to the meal. All of the fruits in Category 1 are so low in energy density that you don't need to worry about limiting portions. You can read more about fruit on page 244.

Protein: I have told you that protein enhances satiety. The protein in the yogurt or milk you add to your high-fiber cereal should be enough to provide this benefit. I know some of you find that boosting your protein at breakfast by eating eggs and lean meats also helps to control hunger. This is okay, just remember to monitor your calories.

While eating breakfast at home is associated with lower body weight, eating restaurant breakfasts regularly is associated with eating more calories and having a higher body weight. If you travel a lot, eat the same healthy breakfast on the road that you do at home. If the restaurant doesn't have what you usually eat, make other healthy choices, such as whole-grain toast or English muffin, oatmeal, fresh fruit, yogurt, or low-fat milk. The breakfast buffet can be a good choice if you go for the cereal and fruit but, if there are a wide variety of choices, you may be tempted to overeat. As with any other meal, you need to be careful about the portions and calories in your breakfast choices.

In this chapter I provide you with recipes for common breakfast foods. Some of the recipes, such as the Mexican Egg Wrap (page 65) or the Piquant Frittata (page 66), also fit well at other meals. You will notice in the menu plan that the weekday breakfast choices are easy to prepare. The options that take more prep time are saved for weekends but, if you have time, go ahead and introduce more variety during the week.

Jennifer's Fruit-Smothered Whole-Wheat Buttermilk Pancakes

Here is a great way for kids to get fruit and fiber. These fresh-fruit-and-raspberry-sauce-topped pancakes are a favorite of my lab manager's son.

1¼ cups whole-wheat flour
1½ cups low-fat buttermilk
1 beaten egg
1 tablespoon sugar
1 teaspoon baking powder

½ teaspoon baking soda
¼ teaspoon salt
½ cup Raspberry Sauce (page 250)
2 cups mixed fresh blueberries,
    raspberries, and blackberries

For a 270-calorie breakfast

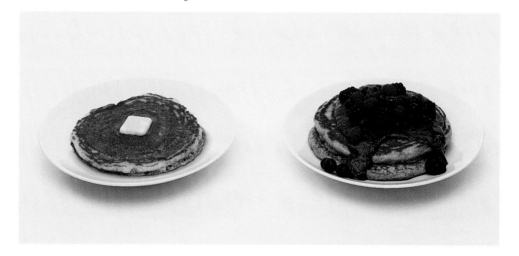

TRADITIONAL	How we lowered the ED	VOLUMETRICS
Pancakes with syrup and butter	▸ Used whole-wheat flour ▸ Omitted oil and butter ▸ Replaced syrup with raspberry sauce ▸ Added fresh fruit	Jennifer's Fruit-Smothered Whole-Wheat Buttermilk Pancakes

1. In a medium mixing bowl, combine the flour, buttermilk, egg, sugar, baking powder, baking soda, and salt. Stir gently until all ingredients are mixed. The batter should be slightly lumpy.

2. Heat a skillet lightly coated with cooking spray over medium heat. Pour ¼ cup batter into the skillet for each pancake. The pancakes will be ready to flip when small bubbles appear along the sides of the pancakes. Flip and cook until the undersides are lightly browned.

3. Place 2 pancakes on each of 4 plates. Spoon 2 tablespoons raspberry sauce over the pancakes and top with ½ cup mixed berries.

YIELD: 4 servings

COOK'S NOTE: Cooked pancakes may be kept warm in a 200 degree oven while you finish cooking the rest.

Nutritional Information Per Serving

Calories 270 | Energy Density 1.0 | Carbohydrate 44 g. | Fat 3 g. | Protein 10 g. | Fiber 8 g.

Baked Berry French Toast

This is an attractive breakfast treat to make on a lazy weekend morning.

1 egg

4 egg whites

1 cup nonfat milk

¼ teaspoon baking powder

½ teaspoon vanilla extract

½ cup sugar

½ teaspoon ground cinnamon

8 ½-inch-thick slices whole-wheat bread

2½ cups frozen unsweetened raspberries

2½ cups frozen sliced unsweetened
  strawberries

1 tablespoon cornstarch

1. Preheat the oven to 400 degrees.

2. Whisk the egg and egg whites lightly in a shallow baking dish. Whisk in the milk, baking powder, vanilla, ¼ cup sugar, and cinnamon. Add the bread, turning to coat. Let the bread stand for 10 minutes, turning occasionally.

3. Lightly coat a 9-by-13-inch baking dish with cooking spray.

4. Combine the frozen berries, ¼ cup sugar, and cornstarch, and spread evenly on the bottom of the baking dish.

5. Arrange the bread slices in a single layer over the berries. Bake until the bread is golden brown and the berries are bubbly, 20 to 25 minutes.

6. Place 2 slices of the French toast and some of the berry mixture on each of 4 plates. Spoon a little of the berry sauce over the toast.

YIELD: 4 servings

COOK'S NOTE: Try other frozen fruit, such as blueberries or peaches. Note that the frozen fruit does not need to be thawed prior to use in this recipe. You may use fresh fruit in place of frozen.

Nutritional Information Per Serving

Calories 315 | Energy Density 1.1 | Carbohydrate 66 g. | Fat 3 g. | Protein 9 g. | Fiber 7 g.

Mexican Egg Wrap

This versatile wrap can be enjoyed at breakfast, lunch, or dinner.

2 slices Canadian bacon, chopped

½ cup shredded zucchini

½ cup diced mushrooms, about 2 ounces

½ cup seeded, diced red or green bell pepper

4 eggs

4 egg whites

¼ teaspoon hot-pepper sauce

Pinch salt

4 flour tortillas

4 tablespoons Cherry Tomato Salsa (page 240)

4 tablespoons reduced-fat shredded Mexican-blend cheese

1. Lightly coat a nonstick skillet with cooking spray and heat over medium heat. Sauté the Canadian bacon for 3 or 4 minutes, until it is browned. Add the zucchini, mushrooms, and bell pepper, and sauté for 2 minutes.

2. In a medium bowl, beat the eggs, egg whites, hot-pepper sauce, and salt. Pour the egg mixture into the pan and scramble with the bacon and vegetables. Cook, stirring frequently, until the eggs are cooked to your liking.

3. Heat the tortillas by steaming them in the microwave in moist paper towels for 20 to 30 seconds.

4. Divide the egg mixture among the tortillas and top with the salsa and cheese. Fold the tortillas in half and serve.

YIELD: 4 servings

COOK'S NOTE: Substitute ¼ cup chopped onion or another vegetable for the Canadian bacon and sauté with the zucchini to create a vegetarian version. Corn tortillas can be used in place of flour tortillas.

Nutritional Information Per Serving

Calories 240 | Energy Density 1.3 | Carbohydrate 21 g. | Fat 9 g. | Protein 17 g. | Fiber 2 g.

Piquant Frittata

Try this egg dish for breakfast along with fresh fruit or have it for lunch with a side salad.

5 whole eggs

7 egg whites

½ teaspoon salt

Freshly ground black pepper

1 cup nonfat shredded mozzarella cheese

1 cup chopped onions

1½ cups sliced mushrooms, about 6 ounces

1 cup diced zucchini

¾ cup chopped bottled roasted red peppers, drained

1 teaspoon dried thyme

3 tablespoons grated Parmesan cheese

For a 175-calorie entrée

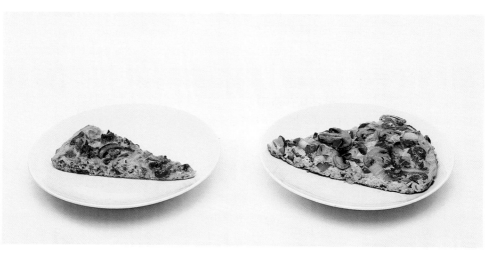

TRADITIONAL	How we lowered the ED	VOLUMETRICS
Frittata with eggs and meat	▸ Reduced number of egg yolks and cheese ▸ Used reduced-fat cheese ▸ Added more vegetables and egg whites ▸ Omitted the meat	Piquant Frittata

1. In a medium bowl, combine the eggs, egg whites, ¼ teaspoon salt, and a few grindings of black pepper and stir in the mozzarella.

2. Lightly coat a large, oven-safe, nonstick skillet with cooking spray and warm over medium heat. Add the onions and mushrooms and cook, stirring, 5 minutes. Add the zucchini, red peppers, thyme, ¼ teaspoon salt, and pinch black pepper. Cook the mixture, stirring, 4 minutes.

3. Pour the egg mixture over the vegetables and cook over medium-high heat for 7 minutes. As the eggs begin to set, run a spatula around the edges and tilt the skillet to allow any uncooked egg to run under the cooked portions. Do not stir. When the eggs are almost set, cover, reduce the heat to medium-low, and cook for 8 to 10 minutes, or until the eggs are set.

4. Preheat the broiler.

5. Sprinkle Parmesan on top of the eggs. Broil the frittata for 4 minutes or until the Parmesan is lightly browned. Cut the frittata into 6 wedges.

YIELD: 6 servings

COOK'S NOTE: Vegetables such as asparagus, broccoli, cauliflower, or yellow summer squash can be substituted for the zucchini.

Nutritional Information Per Serving

Calories 175 | Energy Density 1.0 | Carbohydrate 9 g. | Fat 8 g. | Protein 16 g. | Fiber 1 g.

Blueberry Applesauce Muffins

These fruit-filled muffins work well for breakfast or as a snack. Applesauce replaces most of the fat traditionally used in baking, and helps keep the muffins moist.

1¾ cups all-purpose flour
¾ cup light brown sugar
½ cup whole-wheat flour
2 teaspoons baking powder
1 teaspoon baking soda
¼ teaspoon salt
¼ teaspoon grated nutmeg

1 teaspoon ground cinnamon
1¼ cups low-fat buttermilk
1¼ cups unsweetened applesauce
1 egg
1 teaspoon vegetable oil
1 teaspoon vanilla extract
1½ cups fresh blueberries

1. Preheat the oven to 400 degrees.

2. Lightly coat a 16-cup muffin pan with cooking spray.

3. Mix together 1½ cups all-purpose flour, sugar, whole-wheat flour, baking powder, baking soda, salt, nutmeg, and cinnamon in a large bowl. Make a well in the center of the mixture.

4. Whisk together the buttermilk, applesauce, egg, oil, and vanilla extract in a small bowl.

5. Toss the blueberries in ¼ cup all-purpose flour to lightly coat the berries.

6. Pour the buttermilk mixture into the flour mixture and stir until the batter is just moistened. Fold in the blueberries.

7. Divide the mixture evenly among the muffin cups. Bake the muffins for 20 minutes. Cool the muffins in the pan on a rack for 5 minutes. Remove the muffins and serve warm or at room temperature.

YIELD: 16 servings

COOK'S NOTE: Be sure to use fresh berries, as frozen may make the batter too watery.

Nutritional Information Per Serving

Calories 125 | Energy Density 1.6 | Carbohydrate 25 g. | Fat 1 g. | Protein 3 g. | Fiber 1 g.

Creamy Apricot Oatmeal

This high-fiber cereal makes a hearty and satisfying breakfast.

1½ cups quick-cooking rolled oats

4 cups nonfat milk

½ teaspoon grated nutmeg

4 tablespoons oat bran

10 finely chopped dried apricots, about 2 ounces

2 tablespoons brown sugar

1. Combine the oats and 3 cups milk in a medium saucepan. Bring the mixture to a boil over medium-high heat, stirring. Mix in the nutmeg and oat bran. Reduce the heat to low and simmer, stirring frequently, until the oats are tender, about 1 minute.

2. Divide the oatmeal among 4 cereal bowls. Sprinkle each with the apricots and brown sugar.

3. Serve the oatmeal immediately, with the remaining milk to add to the oatmeal, if desired.

YIELD: 4 servings

COOK'S NOTE: The apricots can be easily chopped using kitchen scissors. Try other dried fruit, such as dried plums, in place of the apricots. The remaining 1 cup milk can be warmed prior to serving.

Nutritional Information Per Serving

Calories 265 | Energy Density 0.90 | Carbohydrate 47 g. | Fat 3 g. | Protein 15 g. | Fiber 5 g.

4 Appetizers, Starters, and Snacks

The types of foods included in this chapter are often intended to give you just a taste of a food or to suppress hunger between meals or until you get to the entrée. The problem is that these foods are often so tasty and come in so many varieties, it is easy to forget portion control. I am going to give you some delicious recipes and tips to help you avoid overeating at parties, before meals, or between meals.

APPETIZERS AND STARTERS

We often begin a meal with appetizers and starters when dining out, or they may be served at parties and receptions to provide something to nibble on while socializing before dinner. When you add an extra course or nibble before a meal, you risk adding extra calories. The variety of tastes, odors, colors, and textures keeps your appetite alive. If you are having appetizers or a starter, you need to budget the calories. In the menu plans (pages 269–271) I will show you how to combine courses over a meal so that you eat the right amount.

When you are dining out or at a party, you need a strategy.

- Don't arrive too hungry. Have a filling snack of fresh fruit or vegetables or a glass of milk before you leave home. This will help you to resist the wide variety of tasty energy-dense options that will tempt you to overeat.

- When asked to bring food to a friend's home or party, take along a volumetric appetizer so you will be sure to have a healthy, low-calorie food to enjoy. Or take a simple dish such as prosciutto with melon. All you need to do is top a slice of ripe melon with thin slices of prosciutto with most of the fat removed, and you have an appetizer with only 120 calories and an energy density of 0.6. Another easy dish is smoked salmon on Belgian endive. Top the endive leaves with a bit of Yogurt Cheese (page 89), smoked salmon, a dash of lemon juice, and a pinch of chopped dill and black pepper. Each leaf has only 25 calories and an energy density of 0.58.
- Variety tempts us to eat more than we need. To manage variety, survey the buffet or selection of appetizers, then fill your plate with veggies and fruit. If there are sauces or dressings, skip them or put a small amount on the side of your plate and use sparingly. Go ahead and sample the foods that look particularly appealing. Take small amounts, then decide whether you need more. If you do, focus on two or three of the choices that you most enjoyed and, again, take small amounts.
- Be aware that seeing food on the plate provides important information about how much you are eating. If you nibble, or keep going back for more, it will be easy to overeat since you are bypassing these visual cues.
- Savor special treats or new recipes. Don't waste calories on energy-dense foods that are available anytime, such as chips.
- Move away from the food so you are less tempted to nibble.
- Slow down on the alcohol. Remember that it adds calories and undermines your resolve to keep your eating under control.
- Hold a glass in your dominant hand. This keeps you away from the finger food, and remember that a glass of water or seltzer works as well as wine or beer.
- Focus on your friends rather than the food.

SNACKS

For many people, eating and drinking between meals adds extra calories to their day. It may be that snacking has become a habit. Even if they are not hungry, they find it is fun to join in when others at work stop for a doughnut midmorning or cookies in the afternoon. The problem is the choice of snacks, not the snacking. Such energy-dense foods are easy to overeat and can quickly add up to 200 to 500 calories, even though 100 calories would be enough to satisfy hunger.

Check your food diary (page 38) to determine what you are eating between meals and where you can make improvements. Studies show that you will eat the same amount at meals whether you snack between meals or not. This does not mean that you should not snack—a small amount between meals can help you to avoid becoming so hungry that you lose control of your intake at mealtime. Be mindful of your hunger (page 40), and eat just enough to satisfy it.

Snacks provide a great opportunity to increase your fruit and vegetable intake. For a filling fruit-based snack, have B's Favorite Smoothie (page 90) or a Tropical Island Smoothie (page 91). Take snacks with you to work. If you know that you have an apple or some yogurt with you, the vending machine will be less tempting. For lots of snack ideas, turn to pages 286–289.

Vegetable Party Platter

Serve this colorful selection of low-energy-dense veggies when you entertain to ensure that you and your guests will have delicious and nutritious nibbles.

2 medium cucumbers, approximately
   1 pound
2 yellow squash, about 1 pound
2 large red bell peppers, about 1 pound
2 large yellow bell peppers, about 1 pound
4 celery stalks
1 pound peeled carrots
1 pound thin asparagus

1 pint small white mushrooms, trimmed
1 pint cherry tomatoes
3 cups broccoli florets
3 cups cauliflowerettes
House Dressing (page 76)
Mel's Fresh Lemon Hummus
   (page 77)
Tex-Mex Salsa (page 78)

1. Cut the cucumbers, squash, bell peppers, celery, and carrots into ¾"-wide x 3-inch-long strips. Trim the asparagus spears and blanch them in boiling water for 4 minutes. Drain, plunge them into ice water for a few minutes, then drain again.

2. Arrange the vegetables on a large platter, placing vegetables of different colors next to each other. Place the house dressing, hummus, and salsa in serving bowls.

YIELD: 16 servings

Nutritional Information Per Serving

Calories 175 | Energy density 0.49 | Carbohydrate 30 g. | Fat 4 g. | Protein 10 g. | Fiber 8 g.

For a 175-calorie appetizer

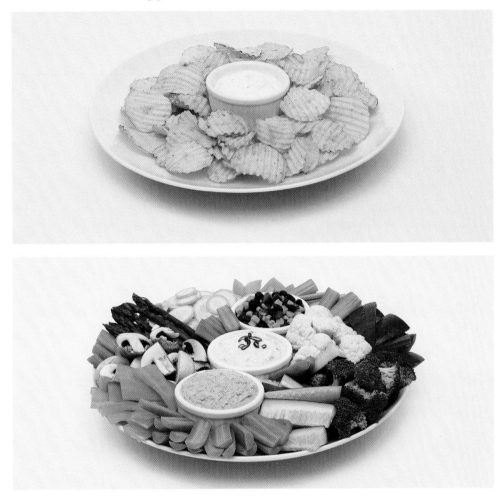

TRADITIONAL	How we lowered the ED	VOLUMETRICS
Chips and dip	▸ Replaced potato chips with vegetables ▸ Substituted low-fat dips for high-fat dips	Vegetable Party Platter

House Dressing

Coriander and cumin give this creamy salad dressing an exotic taste. It is also good as a dip with cut-up fresh vegetables.

½ teaspoon minced garlic

¼ teaspoon salt

2 tablespoons lime juice

½ teaspoon Worcestershire sauce

½ teaspoon ground coriander

½ teaspoon ground cumin

1 tablespoon minced scallions

1 cup Yogurt Cheese (page 89)

1 cup low-fat buttermilk

Pinch freshly ground black pepper

1. Whisk all the ingredients in a large bowl until blended, but still slightly chunky.

YIELD: 24 servings of 2 tablespoons each

Nutritional Information Per Serving

Calories 35 | Energy Density 0.75 | Carbohydrate 4 g. | Fat 1 g. | Protein 3 g. | Fiber 0 g.

Mel's Fresh Lemon Hummus

This tangy hummus, developed by my daughter Melissa, is delicious either as a dip with raw vegetables or as a sandwich filling.

¼ to ⅓ cup freshly squeezed lemon juice

2 cups canned chickpeas, rinsed and drained

¼ cup tahini

2 teaspoons chopped garlic

1 teaspoon grated lemon zest

½ teaspoon salt

1. Puree ¼ cup lemon juice with the rest of the ingredients in a blender or food processor until the texture is slightly chunky. Taste and, if desired, stir in more lemon juice.

YIELD: 10 servings of 2 tablespoons each

Nutritional Information Per Serving

Calories 90 | Energy Density 1.7 | Carbohydrate 13 g. | Fat 3 g. | Protein 3 g. | Fiber 2 g.

Tex-Mex Salsa

Add a Southwestern flair to any meal by using this mild salsa as a garnish for fish or chicken. It can also be used as a topping for baked potatoes or as a dip with raw vegetables.

1¾ cups canned black beans, rinsed and drained

2 cups canned whole-kernel corn, drained

1 cup seeded, chopped red or green bell peppers

½ cup chopped fresh cilantro or fresh flat-leaf parsley

1 cup chopped scallions

3 tablespoons lime juice

2 tablespoons red-wine vinegar

½ teaspoon ground cumin

¼ teaspoon salt

¼ teaspoon hot-pepper sauce

1. Combine all the ingredients in a large bowl. The salsa can be refrigerated for up to 3 days.

YIELD: 8 servings of ½ cup each

COOK'S NOTE: The flavor of this salsa intensifies as the beans and vegetables marinate.

Nutritional Information Per Serving

Calories 95 | Energy Density 0.65 | Carbohydrate 18 g. | Fat 1 g. | Protein 5 g. | Fiber 5 g.

White Bean Bruschetta

Bruschetta (pronounced brew-sketta) is an easy to make appetizer. Just spread a tasty topping on slices of toasted or grilled bread.

2 cups canned cannellini beans,
   rinsed and drained
1 tablespoon lemon juice
1 tablespoon extra-virgin olive oil
1 teaspoon minced garlic
1 tablespoon chopped, fresh flat-leaf
   parsley

1 tablespoon chopped dill
¼ teaspoon salt
16 slices toasted or grilled baguette,
   cut ¼-inch thick on the diagonal
1 garlic clove, cut in half

1. Puree all ingredients except the baguette and the halved garlic clove.

2. Rub both sides of the toasted baguette slices with the cut side of the garlic halves.

3. Spread the bean mixture on the bread slices and serve.

YIELD: 16 servings of 1 toast slice and 1½ tablespoons of bean mixture each

COOK'S NOTE: For another easy topping, combine ¼ cup chopped basil with 2 cups chopped tomatoes, 1 teaspoon minced garlic, 2 teaspoons extra-virgin olive oil, ½ teaspoon salt, and a dash of pepper. Each serving has 45 calories and an energy density of 1.2.

Nutritional Information Per Serving

Calories 60 | Energy Density 1.5 | Carbohydrate 11 g. | Fat 1 g. | Protein 3 g. | Fiber 2 g.

Lemon Shrimp Bruschetta

2 cups shredded arugula

12 slices toasted or grilled baguette, cut
    ¼-inch thick on the diagonal

1 tablespoon extra-virgin olive oil

2 thinly sliced garlic cloves

12 peeled and deveined large shrimp,
    about ½ pound

4 tablespoons lemon juice

¼ cup dry white wine

¼ cup chopped chives

1 tablespoon grated lemon zest

1. Divide the arugula among 4 dinner plates. Place 3 slices of toasted bread on top of each plate of arugula.

2. Lightly coat a large nonstick skillet with cooking spray. Add the oil and heat to almost smoking over medium heat. Add the garlic and stir until light brown, about 1 minute.

3. Add the shrimp to the skillet and cook 2 to 3 minutes, or until bright pink. Turn the shrimp over. Add the lemon juice and wine and cook, stirring, 1 minute. Using a slotted spoon or tongs, place 1 shrimp on each bread slice.

4. Stir the chives into the sauce in the skillet. Spoon the sauce over the shrimp and sprinkle with the lemon zest.

YIELD: 4 servings

COOK'S NOTE: Any lettuce or combination of greens can be used in place of the arugula. Nonfat chicken broth can be used in place of the wine.

Nutritional Information Per Serving

Calories 215 | Energy Density 1.6 | Carbohydrate 22 g. | Fat 6 g. | Protein 16 g. | Fiber 1 g.

Insalata Caprese

The combination of fresh basil and mozzarella enhances the flavor of sweet vine-ripened tomatoes in this simple and colorful first course.

4 medium ripe slicing tomatoes,
   about 1½ pounds
⅓ pound ball fresh mozzarella cheese

4 cups shredded arugula
18 to 20 fresh basil leaves
Balsamic Dressing (page 152)

1. Core and cut each tomato into ¼" slices.

2. Slice the mozzarella into ⅛" thick rounds.

3. Divide the arugula among 6 plates. Arrange the tomato, mozzarella, and basil in overlapping slices on the arugula.

4. Drizzle 1 tablespoon dressing over each salad.

YIELD: 6 servings

COOK'S NOTE: Mixed spring greens can be used in place of the arugula.

Nutritional Information Per Serving

Calories 105 | Energy Density 0.81 | Carbohydrate 6 g. | Fat 7 g. | Protein 6 g. | Fiber 1 g.

Asian Spring Rolls with Soy-Ginger Dipping Sauce

These appetizers will provide an exotic start to your next dinner party.

¼ cup lime juice

¼ cup rice-wine vinegar

1 tablespoon sesame oil

1 tablespoon reduced-sodium soy sauce

2 teaspoons brown sugar

2 teaspoons minced fresh ginger

1 ounce uncooked rice sticks

1 cup peeled, shredded carrots

¼ cup packed fresh cilantro leaves

3 tablespoons shredded fresh basil

1 cup shredded green-leaf lettuce

1 teaspoon chopped garlic

¼ cup finely chopped scallions

¼ teaspoon crushed red-pepper flakes

1 cup seeded, chopped, red bell peppers

16 cooked medium shrimp, shelled and deveined, about ⅔ pound unshelled

8 8-inch-round rice-paper sheets

For a 130-calorie appetizer

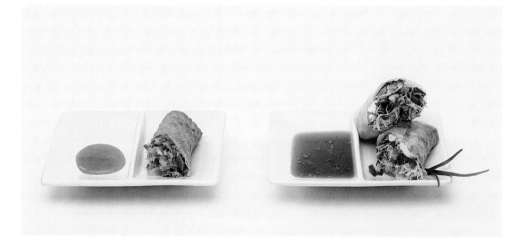

TRADITIONAL	How we lowered the ED	VOLUMETRICS
Egg rolls	▸ Used a thinner wrapper ▸ Served fresh instead of fried	Asian Spring Rolls

1. Place the lime juice, vinegar, oil, soy sauce, sugar, and ginger in a screw-top jar. Shake vigorously until blended. Set the Soy-Ginger Dipping Sauce aside.

2. Bring 1 quart of water to a boil. Add the rice sticks, cook for 3 minutes. Drain, run under cold water, drain again.

3. Combine the rice sticks, carrots, cilantro, basil, lettuce, garlic, scallions, red-pepper flakes, and bell peppers in a large bowl.

4. Cut each shrimp in half lengthwise.

5. Place one rice-paper sheet in a shallow bowl or pan. Cover with 1" hot water and let stand for 30 seconds, or until soft. Place the sheet on a flat work surface.

6. Place ½ cup rice-stick filling in the center of the sheet. Arrange 4 shrimp pieces on the filling.

7. Fold in both sides and then the bottom of the sheet over the filling. Then roll it up from the bottom to close. Gently press the seam to seal. Place the roll on a plate and cover with a damp towel.

8. Repeat with the remaining rice-paper sheets, filling, and shrimp.

9. Place the Soy-Ginger Dipping Sauce in a small bowl and serve with the rolls.

YIELD: 8 servings of 1 spring roll with 1 tablespoon sauce

COOK'S NOTE: Rice sticks, rice-paper sheets, rice-wine vinegar, sesame oil, and soy sauce are available in the international section of large supermarkets and in Asian specialty stores. Substitute sliced mushrooms or cucumber for the shrimp to create a vegetarian version.

Nutritional Information Per Serving

Calories 130 | Energy Density 1.2 | Carbohydrate 15 g. | Fat 1 g. | Protein 13 g. | Fiber 1 g.

Nutritional Information Per Serving of Sauce Alone

Calories 25 | Energy Density 1.2 | Carbohydrate 2 g. | Fat 2 g. | Protein 0 g. | Fiber 1 g.

Sesame Mushroom Kebobs

Try these Asian-inspired kebobs as a vegetarian appetizer when you are grilling.

12 ounces white mushrooms

2 bunches large scallions, about 10

2 bell peppers, any color, seeded and cut
   into 1½-inch squares, about 1 pound

¼ cup reduced-sodium soy sauce

2 tablespoons sugar

1 tablespoon sesame oil

4 teaspoons minced garlic

2 tablespoons toasted sesame seeds
   (see Cook's Note)

½ teaspoon freshly ground black pepper

1. Trim the mushroom stems and cut mushroom caps into ½" thick slices. Trim and cut the white parts of scallions into 1½" pieces. Trim and finely chop enough scallion greens tops to make ¼ cup. Set aside.

2. Thread the mushroom slices onto 6 skewers so that they will lie flat on the grill, alternating with scallion whites and bell pepper squares, threaded crosswise. Arrange the skewers in a baking dish that will hold them snugly.

3. In a small bowl, whisk the soy sauce, sugar, oil, garlic, 1 tablespoon sesame seeds, and black pepper. Pour this marinade over the skewers, turning to coat all sides. Cover and marinate for 30 minutes or up to 2 hours, turning once.

4. Preheat the grill or broiler to high. Place the skewers on the rack and cook, brushing often with the marinade, for 3 to 5 minutes per side, or until browned.

5. Remove the skewers and sprinkle with 1 tablespoon of the sesame seeds and the scallion greens. Serve with any remaining marinade as a dipping sauce.

YIELD: 6 servings

COOK'S NOTE: To toast seeds or nuts, place in a skillet, and cook over moderate heat, stirring, until golden.

Nutritional Information Per Serving

Calories 90 | Energy Density 0.70 | Carbohydrate 11 g. | Fat 4 g. | Protein 4 g. | Fiber 2 g.

Mushroom and Cheese Quesadillas with Mango Salsa

Try these to start a Southwestern-inspired meal. Quesadillas are also popular as a main course for lunch or dinner—just double the serving size.

½ teaspoon salt

1 teaspoon vegetable oil

5 cups thinly sliced, mixed mushrooms (white, portobello and shiitake), about 1 pound

½ cup finely chopped onions

1 cup seeded, chopped red bell peppers

1 teaspoon minced garlic

⅛ teaspoon freshly ground black pepper

8 6-inch flour tortillas

½ cup shredded reduced-fat Monterey Jack cheese

Mango Salsa (page 88)

1. Heat the oil in a large skillet coated with cooking spray over medium-high heat. Add the mushrooms and cook, stirring, 2 minutes. Remove 1 cup mushrooms and set aside.

2. Add the onions, bell peppers, garlic, salt, and black pepper. Cook, stirring, 3 to 4 minutes, or until the liquid evaporates.

3. Divide the mushroom mixture among 4 tortillas. Divide the Monterey Jack over the mushroom mixture and top with the remaining tortillas.

4. Clean the skillet with paper towels and heat over medium-high heat. Add 1 quesadilla, press down lightly with a spatula, and cook for about 1 minute, turning once, or until lightly browned. Remove from the skillet and keep warm. Repeat with the remaining quesadillas.

5. Cut each quesadilla into 4 wedges, distribute among 8 plates, and top with the reserved mushroom mixture and the Mango Salsa.

YIELD: 8 servings

Nutritional Information Per Serving

Calories 175 | Energy Density 1.4 | Carbohydrate 23 g. | Fat 5 g. | Protein 6 g. | Fiber 3 g.

Stuffed Mushrooms Florentine

These appetizers are low in calories and fat yet packed with flavor. Present them with other appetizers such as the Vegetable Party Platter (page 74) at your next party.

12 large white mushrooms, about 1½ inches across
1 teaspoon vegetable oil
¾ cup minced onions
½ teaspoon minced garlic
½ cup finely chopped spinach

½ cup seeded finely chopped red or green bell peppers
1 tablespoon fresh thyme
¼ teaspoon salt
Pinch freshly ground black pepper
1 tablespoon grated Parmesan cheese

For a 45-calorie appetizer

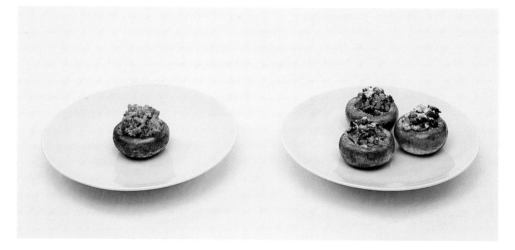

TRADITIONAL	How we lowered the ED	VOLUMETRICS
Sausage-stuffed mushrooms	▸ Omitted sausage ▸ Added vegetables ▸ Decreased cheese	Stuffed Mushrooms Florentine

1. Remove, trim, and finely chop the mushroom stems, set aside.

2. Bring a medium pot of water to a boil. Blanch the mushroom caps for 2 minutes. Remove the caps and place gill side down on paper towels to drain.

3. Lightly coat a medium nonstick skillet with cooking spray, add the oil, and place over medium heat until hot. Add the reserved mushroom stems and the rest of the ingredients except the cheese, and cook, stirring occasionally, for 6 minutes. Remove the skillet from the heat and cool slightly.

4. Preheat the broiler.

5. Spoon the mixture into the mushroom caps and place on a baking sheet. Sprinkle with Parmesan. Broil the mushroom caps until light brown, about 3 minutes.

YIELD: 4 servings of 3 mushroom caps each

COOK'S NOTE: This appetizer may be frozen before broiling. When ready to proceed, thaw the mushrooms and broil as directed.

Nutritional Information Per Serving

Calories 45 | Energy Density 0.40 | Carbohydrate 5 g. | Fat 3 g. | Protein 3 g. | Fiber 2 g.

Guacamole

This traditional Mexican dip can also be used as a sandwich spread.

2 ripe avocados, peeled and pitted
2 tablespoons lime juice
⅛ teaspoon salt
¼ cup chopped fresh cilantro

½ cup chopped onions
1 cup cored chopped tomatoes
¼ teaspoon minced garlic
¼ teaspoon hot-pepper sauce

1. In a medium bowl, mash the avocados with the lime juice and salt. Stir in the cilantro, onions, tomatoes, garlic, and hot-pepper sauce. Cover with plastic wrap and refrigerate for 1 hour before serving.

YIELD: 12 servings of 2 tablespoons each

Nutritional Information Per Serving

Calories 65 | Energy Density 0.83 | Carbohydrate 6 g. | Fat 5 g. | Protein 1 g. | Fiber 3 g.

Mango Salsa

2 cups diced mango
3 tablespoons lime juice
2 tablespoons chopped cilantro

1 tablespoon finely chopped jalapeno
¼ teaspoon salt

1. In a small bowl, combine the mango, lime juice, cilantro, jalapeno, and ¼ teaspoon salt.

YIELD: 4 servings

COOK'S NOTE: Fresh Peaches can be substituted for the mango.

Nutritional Information Per Serving

Calories 58 | Energy Density 0.6 | Carbohydrate 15 g. | Fat 0 g. | Protein 0 g. | Fiber 2 g.

Yogurt Cheese

This alternative to regular cream cheese has no fat. Use it as a spread for toast or to top baked potatoes.

3 cups nonfat plain yogurt

1. Set a fine-mesh sieve or colander over a bowl. Line it with a double layer of cheesecloth. Spoon in the yogurt and cover the bowl with plastic wrap. Refrigerate for at least 8 hours or overnight. Transfer the yogurt cheese to a covered storage container and discard the liquid.

YIELD: 16 servings of 1 tablespoon each, about 1 cup total

COOK'S NOTE: The yogurt cheese will keep in the refrigerator for up to 1 week. You can vary the flavor by adding fresh chopped herbs, minced garlic, and/or lemon zest. Begin with small amounts, adjusting to taste.

Nutritional Information Per Serving

Calories 15 | Energy Density 0.90 | Carbohydrate 2 g. | Fat 0 g. | Protein 2 g. | Fiber 0 g.

B's Favorite Smoothie

This is one of my favorite snacks. Volumetric smoothies, with lots of fruit and little fat, are particularly satisfying.

3 cups crushed ice

1 cup sliced fresh or frozen strawberries

1 medium banana, peeled and sliced

1 cup nonfat, sugarfree, strawberry yogurt

1. Place all the ingredients in a blender. Puree until smooth, approximately 1 minute.

2. Distribute among 4 glasses and serve immediately.

YIELD: 4 servings

COOK'S NOTE: Any fresh or frozen berries and other flavors of yogurt may be used.

Nutritional Information Per Serving

Calories 80 | Energy Density 0.42 | Carbohydrate 17 g. | Fat 0 g. | Protein 3 g. | Fiber 2 g.

For an 80-calorie snack

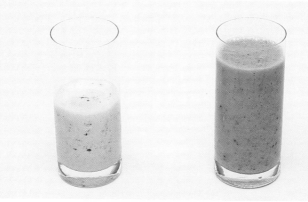

TRADITIONAL	How we lowered the ED	VOLUMETRICS
Strawberry milkshake	▸ Used nonfat, sugarfree yogurt instead of whole milk and ice cream ▸ Used plenty of fresh fruit ▸ Added ice to increase volume without adding calories	B's Favorite Smoothie

Tropical Island Smoothie

1 cup crushed ice

1 cup coconut sorbet

2 cups fresh pineapple cubes

1½ cups peeled, pitted, diced fresh mango

1. Place all the ingredients in a blender. Puree until smooth, approximately 1 minute.

2. Distribute among 4 glasses and serve immediately.

YIELD: 4 servings

COOK'S NOTE: Drained, canned pineapple can be substituted for the fresh pineapple.

Nutritional Information Per Serving

Calories 165 | Energy Density 0.70 | Carbohydrate 39 g. | Fat 2 g. | Protein 1 g. | Fiber 2 g.

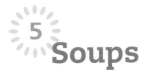

5 Soups

We know more about soup and satiety than we do any other type of food. The high water content and low energy density make it naturally filling. In addition, other high-satiety, nutritious ingredients such as lean protein and fiber-rich vegetables and grains can be combined in soups. Be careful! Some soups, such as those that are cream-based, can be loaded with calories.

I have shown in several studies that eating a broth-based soup before a meal fills you up, so that you eat less of the main course. As with any first course, you must make sure the calories are not too high—aim for 150 calories or less. Go higher, and you may end up consuming more total calories at the meal. To help fill you up, keep the volume high. You can do this by adding water and low-calorie veggies. No, I am not asking you to eat watery, unappealing soups. With the recipes in this chapter I show you how you can have soups that do it all—they are nutritious, tasty, and filling.

By the way, this raises a question I suspect you have been asking. That is, if you eat less at a meal because you filled up on a food like soup that is low in energy density, won't you just get hungry sooner? We have not seen that in our studies. Our bodies are just not that sensitive to calories. So, if you save 100 calories at lunch by eating soup, you are unlikely to feel hungrier at dinner. In our studies, people did not make up for the calories saved at lunch by eating more at dinner.

So, go for soup as a first course, a snack, or a meal. It is a proven way to control hunger and manage your weight. Here are some helpful tips:

- Start your meal with a low-energy-dense soup. If you increase the volume by adding water or water-rich ingredients, you will feel fuller and eat less of the main course. Some low-calorie, low-energy-dense options are Minestrone (page 102 and Gazpacho (page 110).
- Make a meal of soup. To ensure that you get a good variety of nutrients and feel satiated, choose soups that have lean meat or beans along with the veggies and broth. I have included several soups that make a nutritious and filling meal, for example, try Asian Black Bean Soup (page 104) or Hearty Chicken and Vegetable Soup (page 108).
- Grab soup for a snack, but keep the calories low: 100 calories if you are just a little hungry, or 200 calories if you have a big case of the munchies.
- If making your own soup, it is okay to use canned or frozen vegetables and cans of broth for convenience—when using broth, choose a nonfat or low-fat, reduced-sodium version. Add herbs for flavor, and small amounts of salt to taste.
- Make large batches of soup and freeze in single servings you can microwave later.
- There are many tasty, convenient, and inexpensive ready-to-eat soups available that can be a snack or part of a meal. Just make sure you check the label—some cans contain more than one serving and may have more calories than you need.
- Add extra fresh or frozen veggies to your soup. This lowers the energy density and adds more texture as well as fiber and nutrients.
- Beware of sneaky calories in soup, especially when eating out. Before ordering, ask how the soup is prepared. If it is cream-based or has lots of butter or oil, it is likely to be high in calories.

Corn and Tomato Chowder

This rich-tasting soup is thickened with potatoes instead of cream.

1 teaspoon unsalted butter
1 cup chopped onions
1 cup chopped celery
3 cups peeled, diced, boiling potatoes
1 bay leaf
2 cups nonfat, reduced-sodium chicken
  broth

1½ cups canned diced tomatoes,
  with liquid
1½ cups frozen corn, thawed
1½ cups nonfat milk
Freshly ground black pepper
½ cup chopped, fresh flat-leaf
  parsley

1. Lightly spray a 4- to 5-quart nonstick pot with cooking spray. Add the butter and place over medium heat. Add the onions and cook, stirring, 5 minutes. Add the celery and potatoes and cook, stirring occasionally, for 2 minutes.

2. Add the bay leaf and broth and bring to a simmer. Cover the pot and cook 20 minutes, stirring occasionally to prevent sticking.

3. Remove the bay leaf, puree 2 cups soup in a blender or food processor, and return to the pot.

4. Stir in the tomatoes, corn, and milk. Return the soup to a simmer, stirring, and cook for 5 minutes, stirring occasionally.

5. Stir in a few grindings of the black pepper, ladle the soup into 8 soup bowls, and serve, garnished with parsley.

YIELD: 8 servings of 1 cup each

COOK'S NOTE: Fresh corn kernels can also be used. Substitute 1 cup vegetable broth and 1 cup of water for the chicken broth to make this a vegetarian soup. This soup freezes well.

Nutritional Information Per Serving

Calories 105 | Energy Density 0.40 | Carbohydrate 19 g. | Fat 2 g. | Protein 5 g. | Fiber 2 g.

Autumn Harvest Pumpkin Soup

Start a meal with this low-fat, beautifully colored soup enlivened with cumin.

2 teaspoons unsalted butter
2 cups chopped onions
2 teaspoons all-purpose flour
4 cups nonfat, reduced-sodium chicken broth
3 cups plain pumpkin puree

½ teaspoon minced garlic
½ teaspoon ground cumin
¼ teaspoon salt
¼ teaspoon ground white pepper
4 tablespoons nonfat plain yogurt
Dusting of grated nutmeg

For a 150-calorie soup

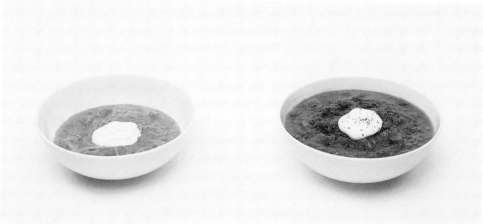

TRADITIONAL	How we lowered the ED	VOLUMETRICS
Pumpkin soup with cream, butter, and sour cream	▸ Substituted broth for cream, and yogurt for sour cream ▸ Decreased butter	Autumn Harvest Pumpkin Soup

1. Lightly coat a 4- to 5-quart nonstick saucepan or pot with cooking spray. Add the butter and place over medium heat. Add the onions and cook, stirring occasionally, 5 minutes.

2. Sprinkle in the flour and cook, stirring, 2 minutes, or until the mixture thickens slightly. Add the broth, whisking, then the pumpkin, garlic, cumin, salt, and pepper. Bring the soup to a simmer, whisking occasionally, and cook 15 minutes, stirring occasionally to prevent scorching.

3. Ladle the soup into 4 soup bowls and top with the yogurt and nutmeg.

YIELD: 4 servings of ⅔ cup each

COOK'S NOTE: Ground coriander can be substituted for cumin. Try adding a teaspoon of grated fresh ginger for extra zip. This can become a vegetarian soup by substituting 2 cups vegetable broth and 2 cups water for the chicken broth.

Nutritional Information Per Serving

Calories 150 | Energy Density 0.40 | Carbohydrate 26 g. | Fat 3 g. | Protein 8 g. | Fiber 7 g.

Creamy Broccoli Soup

2 tablespoons unsalted butter

¾ cup chopped onions

2 tablespoons all-purpose flour

1 teaspoon dry mustard

½ teaspoon dried tarragon

Pinch ground white pepper

2 cups nonfat milk

2 cups nonfat, reduced-sodium chicken broth

4 cups chopped broccoli florets

For a 160-calorie soup

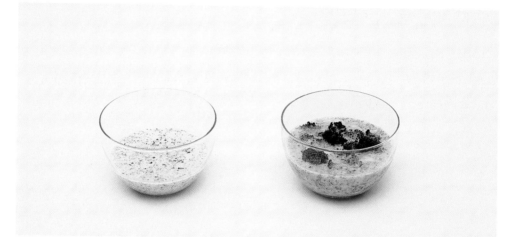

TRADITIONAL	How we lowered the ED	VOLUMETRICS
Broccoli cheese soup	▸ Omitted cheese ▸ Used nonfat milk and chicken broth and less butter ▸ Added more broccoli	Creamy Broccoli Soup

1. Heat the butter in a 4- to 5-quart nonstick pot over medium heat. Add the onions and cook, stirring occasionally, 5 minutes.

2. Raise the heat to medium-high and stir in the flour, mustard, tarragon, and pepper and cook 2 minutes. Reduce the heat to medium. Add the milk and broth and cook, stirring frequently, 8 minutes.

3. Add the broccoli and simmer 6 minutes, stirring frequently. Remove from the heat.

4. Puree 2 cups of soup in a blender or food processor and return to the pot. Reheat, stirring occasionally, about 2 minutes.

YIELD: 4 servings of 1 cup each

COOK'S NOTE: To create a vegetarian version, substitute 1 cup vegetable broth and 1 cup water for the chicken broth.

Nutritional Information Per Serving

Calories 160 | Energy Density 0.60 | Carbohydrate 15 g. | Fat 8 g. | Protein 9 g. | Fiber 2 g.

Curried Cauliflower Soup

This light vegetarian soup makes a delicious first course. The curry complements the cauliflower to create a unique flavor that will add variety to your meals.

1 tablespoon extra-virgin olive oil
1½ cups halved and sliced onions
1 teaspoon curry powder
2 cups vegetable broth

4 cups chopped cauliflowerettes
½ teaspoon salt
2 cups shredded zucchini, about 2 small

1. Heat the oil in a 4- to 5-quart pot over medium heat. Add the onions and curry powder. Cover and cook 4 minutes, stirring occasionally.

2. Add the broth, cauliflower, salt, and 2 cups water to the pot. Bring the soup to a simmer, stirring occasionally. Cover the pot and simmer 15 minutes, stirring occasionally.

3. Puree the soup in a blender or food processor and return to the pot.

4. Reserve 2 tablespoons of the zucchini. Stir the rest of the zucchini into the soup and reheat.

5. Ladle the soup into 4 soup bowls and garnish with the reserved zucchini.

YIELD: 4 servings of 1½ cups each

Nutritional Information Per Serving

Calories 105 | Energy Density 0.30 | Carbohydrate 15 g. | Fat 4 g. | Protein 5 g. | Fiber 4 g.

Rustic Tomato Soup

This Tuscan country soup provides you with a delicious way to use day-old crusty bread. Pictured on page 56.

1 teaspoon extra-virgin olive oil
½ cup chopped onions
½ teaspoon chopped garlic
1½ cups canned diced tomatoes,
    with liquid
½ teaspoon dried oregano
¼ teaspoon salt

1½ cups nonfat, reduced-sodium chicken
    broth
Pinch freshly ground black pepper
4 toasted or grilled baguette slices, cut
    ¼-inch thick on the diagonal
Parmesan cheese shavings

1. Lightly coat a 4- to 5-quart pot with cooking spray. Add the oil and place over medium heat. Stir in the onions and garlic and cook 5 minutes, stirring often. Stir in the tomatoes, oregano, salt, and broth. Bring the soup to a simmer and cook uncovered, 20 minutes, stirring occasionally. Remove from the heat and stir in the pepper.

2. Place 1 slice of toasted bread in the bottom of each of 4 wide, shallow soup bowls. Ladle the soup over the bread. Top with a few shavings of Parmesan.

YIELD: 4 servings of 1½ cups each

COOK'S NOTE: When available, fresh basil makes a delicious addition to the soup. Stir in ½ cup chopped basil with the pepper. Tuscans traditionally use fresh vine-ripened tomatoes for this soup. For a vegetarian version, substitute 1 cup vegetable broth and ½ cup water for the chicken broth.

Nutritional Information Per Serving

Calories 125 | Energy Density 0.40 | Carbohydrate 20 g. | Fat 3 g. | Protein 5 g. | Fiber 3 g.

Minestrone

Pair this vegetarian soup with a sandwich for lunch.

2 teaspoons extra-virgin olive oil

1 cup chopped onions

1 cup peeled, shredded carrots

1½ cups low-sodium vegetable juice

3 cups vegetable broth

1¼ cups cored, diced tomatoes

¾ teaspoon dried thyme

1 teaspoon dried oregano

Freshly ground black pepper

12 ounces dry, whole-wheat small pasta shells, or other whole-wheat small pasta shapes

1 cup canned cannellini beans, rinsed and drained

3 cups shredded fresh spinach

For a 125-calorie soup

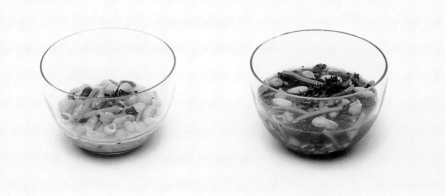

TRADITIONAL	How we lowered the ED	VOLUMETRICS
Cream-based vegetable soup	▸ Decreased oil ▸ Omitted cream ▸ Added more veggies	Minestrone

1. Heat the oil in a 4- to 5-quart pan over medium heat. Add the onions and carrots and cook 5 minutes, stirring occasionally.

2. Add 1 cup water, vegetable juice, broth, tomatoes, thyme, oregano, and a few grindings of pepper. Bring the soup to a boil, reduce the heat, and simmer, covered, 30 minutes.

3. Prepare the pasta according to package directions.

4. Add the cooked pasta, beans, and spinach and cook over medium-low heat for 10 minutes.

YIELD: 8 servings of 1 cup each

COOK'S NOTE: For additional flavor and texture, try adding one of the following: 2 cups shredded cabbage, 2 cups sliced mushrooms, or 1 cup shredded zucchini when adding the spinach.

Nutritional Information Per Serving

Calories 125 | Energy Density 0.50 | Carbohydrate 23 g. | Fat 2 g. | Protein 6 g. | Fiber 4.5 g.

Asian Black Bean Soup

Garlic, soy sauce, and red-pepper flakes give this soup an Asian flair. Pair this soup with a salad for a filling lunch.

2 teaspoons vegetable oil

1 cup chopped onions

2 teaspoons chopped garlic

1 cup nonfat, reduced-sodium chicken broth

3 cups canned black beans, rinsed and drained

2 tablespoons reduced-sodium soy sauce

⅛ teaspoon crushed red-pepper flakes

⅛ teaspoon ground coriander

2 tablespoons orange juice

4 tablespoons reduced-fat sour cream

2 tablespoons chopped scallions

1. Heat the oil in a 4- to 5-quart pot over medium heat. Add the onions and garlic and cook 5 minutes, stirring occasionally. Add the broth, beans, soy sauce, red-pepper flakes, coriander, and ¾ cup water. Bring the soup to a boil, reduce the heat, and simmer, uncovered, 20 minutes.

2. Puree about three-quarters of the soup in a blender or food processor until smooth. Return the pureed soup to the pot and stir in the orange juice. Simmer the soup 5 minutes.

3. Divide the soup among 4 bowls and serve topped with the sour cream and scallions.

YIELD: 4 servings of 1½ cups each

COOK'S NOTE: Serve the soup over ½ cup boiled brown rice for a more substantial meal. Substitute ½ cup vegetable broth and ½ cup water for the chicken broth to make this a vegetarian soup.

Nutritional Information Per Serving

Calories 240 | Energy Density 0.70 | Carbohydrate 32 g. | Fat 6 g. | Protein 13 g. | Fiber 11 g.

Cannellini Bean Soup

This quick and delicious main dish soup will help you to boost your fiber intake.

1 teaspoon extra-virgin olive oil

1 cup chopped onions

1½ teaspoons chopped garlic

2 cups cored, diced tomatoes

2 cups canned cannellini beans, rinsed and drained

1 cup diced zucchini

½ cup frozen peas, thawed

1 cup peeled, thinly sliced carrots

1 tablespoon chopped, fresh flat-leaf parsley

¾ teaspoon dried thyme

Pinch freshly ground black pepper

2 cups vegetable broth

4 tablespoons grated Parmesan cheese

1. Lightly spray a 4- to 5-quart pot with cooking spray and place over medium heat. Add the oil, onions, and garlic and cook 5 minutes, stirring frequently.

2. Stir in 1 cup water and the rest of the ingredients, except the Parmesan. Bring to a simmer, stirring occasionally. Simmer the soup 10 minutes, stirring occasionally.

3. Ladle into 4 soup bowls and sprinkle with Parmesan.

YIELD: 4 servings of 1½ cups each

COOK'S NOTE: Any white bean can be substituted for the cannellini. This soup freezes well.

Nutritional Information Per Serving

Calories 265 | Energy Density 0.50 | Carbohydrate 44 g. | Fat 4 g. | Protein 15 g. | Fiber 10 g.

Lentil and Tomato Soup

Lentils provide an inexpensive source of protein. Combine this nonfat soup with a salad or half-sandwich for a lunch or dinner meal.

1 cup dried lentils
½ teaspoon salt
2 teaspoons chopped garlic
¾ cup chopped onions
¾ cup chopped celery
¾ cup peeled, chopped carrots
¼ teaspoon dried thyme

¼ teaspoon dried oregano
¼ teaspoon freshly ground black pepper
2½ cups canned diced tomatoes, with liquid
1 tablespoon red-wine vinegar
4 tablespoons nonfat sour cream

1. Place the lentils, salt, and 3 cups water in a 4- to 5-quart pot. Bring to a simmer and cook, partially covered, 20 minutes.

2. Stir in the garlic, onions, celery, carrots, thyme, oregano, and pepper and simmer, partially covered, 25 minutes.

3. Stir in the tomatoes and simmer, partially covered, 15 minutes. Stir in the vinegar.

4. Divide the soup among 4 bowls and top with sour cream.

YIELD: 4 servings of 1½ cups each

Nutritional Information Per Serving

Calories 230 | Energy Density 0.60 | Carbohydrate 41 g. | Fat 0 g. | Protein 16 g. | Fiber 17 g.

Vegetarian Barley Soup

Barley provides interesting texture, a nutlike flavor, and lots of nutrients. Serve this soup as part of lunch or dinner.

½ cup chopped onions

¼ cup chopped celery

1 tablespoon chopped, fresh flat-leaf parsley

½ teaspoon chopped garlic

3½ cups vegetable broth

1½ cups canned diced tomatoes, with liquid

½ cup peeled, sliced carrots

¼ cup pearl barley

¼ teaspoon salt

Pinch freshly ground black pepper

¼ teaspoon dried oregano

¼ teaspoon dried thyme

1 bay leaf

2 cups chopped mushrooms, about 6 ounces

1. Coat the bottom of a large Dutch oven or pot with cooking spray and place over medium-high heat until hot. Add the onions, celery, parsley, and garlic and cook, stirring frequently, 4 minutes.

2. Add the broth, tomatoes, carrots, barley, salt, pepper, oregano, thyme, and bay leaf and bring to a simmer, stirring occasionally. Cover the pot and simmer 20 minutes, stirring occasionally.

3. Stir in the mushrooms and simmer, uncovered, 20 minutes, stirring occasionally.

4. Remove and discard the bay leaf. Ladle the soup into 4 bowls.

YIELD: 4 servings of 1¼ cups each

COOK'S NOTE: Try different types of mushrooms to vary the flavor.

Nutritional Information Per Serving

Calories 120 | Energy Density 0.40 | Carbohydrate 19 g. | Fat 2 g. | Protein 8 g. | Fiber 4 g.

Hearty Chicken and Vegetable Soup

Whole-wheat pasta adds fiber to this satisfying main dish soup.

2 tablespoons all-purpose flour
½ teaspoon salt
½ teaspoon dried tarragon
3 4- to 6-ounce skinless, boneless chicken
   breast halves, cut into ½-inch pieces
2 teaspoons vegetable oil
3 cups peeled, chopped carrots
3 cups quartered, small mushrooms,
   about ½ pound

4 cups nonfat, reduced-sodium chicken
   broth
1 teaspoon hot-pepper sauce
4 ounces dry, whole-wheat chiocciole or
   other small whole-wheat pasta
¼ cup chopped, fresh flat-leaf parsley

1. Combine the flour, salt, and tarragon in a large bowl. Add the chicken and toss to coat.

2. Lightly coat the bottom of a 4- to 5-quart pot with cooking spray. Add the oil and place over medium-high heat. Add the chicken and cook, stirring frequently, 5 minutes, or until lightly browned and no longer pink inside. Remove the chicken and set aside.

3. Stir in the carrots, mushrooms, broth, and hot-pepper sauce and bring to a simmer. Cover and simmer 15 minutes, stirring occasionally.

4. Stir in the chiocciole and reserved chicken and cook 12 minutes. Ladle into 4 soup bowls and sprinkle with parsley.

YIELD: 4 servings of 2 cups each

COOK'S NOTE: Two cups of boiled brown rice may be substituted for the pasta. Stir in the rice with the chicken in step 4, cook 5 minutes, and serve as directed above.

Nutritional Information Per Serving

Calories 290 | Energy Density 0.60 | Carbohydrate 37 g. | Fat 7 g. | Protein 24 g. | Fiber 5 g.

For a 290-calorie soup

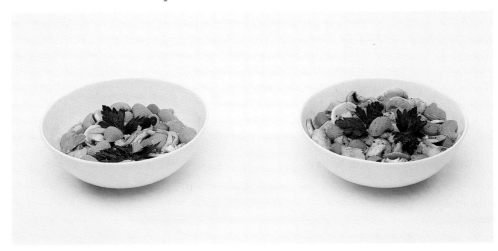

TRADITIONAL	How we lowered the ED	VOLUMETRICS
Chicken and vegetable soup	▸ Used lean, white chicken meat ▸ Decreased oil and pasta ▸ Increased the amount of veggies	Hearty Chicken and Vegetable Soup

Gazpacho

Serve this zesty, chunky version of the traditional Spanish cold soup as a starter.

3 cups cored, chopped tomatoes, about 1½ pounds

1 cup seeded, peeled, chopped cucumber

1 cup chopped green bell peppers

2 jalapenos, seeded and finely chopped

1 cup chopped sweet onions

½ cup chopped celery

1 teaspoon minced garlic

2 cups reduced-sodium vegetable juice

2 tablespoons white-wine vinegar

2 teaspoons extra-virgin olive oil

1 teaspoon hot-pepper sauce

¼ teaspoon salt

¼ teaspoon freshly ground black pepper

1. Place all the ingredients in a large bowl. Stir well. Cover soup and chill 2 hours.

YIELD: 4 servings of 1⅔ cups each

COOK'S NOTE: If you use a food processor to chop the vegetables, process them separately to avoid overprocessing.

Nutritional Information Per Serving

Calories 120 | Energy Density 0.30 | Carbohydrate 19 g. | Fat 3 g. | Protein 5 g. | Fiber 5 g.

6 Sandwiches and Wraps

Sandwiches have been a lunchtime favorite for years. They continue to evolve as creative cooks experiment and restaurants discover that customers are willing to try new combinations. Perhaps you, too, can come up with your own signature sandwich or wrap, but let's make sure you know how to make it volumetric.

One of the first decisions you will make is how big the sandwich or wrap should be. Studies in my lab show that if you choose a large, energy-dense sandwich, you are likely to eat more. Women ate 31 percent more (160 calories) when served a 12-inch submarine sandwich than when served a 6-inch sandwich. Men responded even more to the increase in size, eating 56 percent more (355 calories). So, don't order or make a large sandwich that is packed with energy-dense fillings. If you see more, you are likely to eat more. You are less likely to overeat if you reduce the energy density by bulking up your sandwich with low-calorie ingredients, such as your favorite vegetables. Also remember that the calories from thick-cut bread, mounds of cheese and meat, and fatty spreads can add up quickly, so you need to consider all of the ingredients in sandwiches and wraps.

Think of sandwiches and wraps as a convenient way to package nutritious fillings. Let's start by considering how to make the package volumetric.

- You have heard it already—to boost your intake of fiber and nutrients, you should look for whole grains. Whole-grain breads, buns, bagels, pita, English muffins, and tortillas are available. Remember to check the label to ensure that the whole grains are listed as the first ingredient.

- Look for bread that is sliced thin—you can find this in presliced loaves or you can buy an unsliced loaf and use a bread knife to slice your own.
- Eat your sandwich open-faced. This is traditional for hot roast beef and turkey and even toasted cheese, but it works for any sandwich. You will probably need a knife and fork! Test this option by trying the Open-Faced Roast Beef Sandwich (page 118).
- Buns, bagels, pita, and tortillas come in a variety of sizes. Choose the smallest and you will end up with a reasonable portion.
- Avoid fatty options, such as croissant, cheese bread, focaccia, or bread coated with oil.

Now that you have the package, let's consider what you should put in it.

- Choose vegetables. Lettuce, tomato, and onion are fine, but there is a lot of room for creativity. Add water-packed artichoke hearts, roasted red peppers, raw bell peppers of any color, grated carrot, celery, cucumber, or some avocado.
- Try portobello mushrooms instead of meat. Cook the mushrooms with a small amount of oil and you will have rich, meaty flavor with a lower energy density and fewer calories. To see how delicious this can be, try the Roasted Portobello Sandwich (page 119).
- If you like cheese, try to use less, or find low-fat versions of cheeses that you like. If you use cheese with a strong flavor, such as aged Cheddar, Swiss, or Gruyere, you will be able to reduce the amount you use without compromising taste.
- When choosing meat, you know what to do—be careful with the amount of choices like fried chicken and other higher-fat options like salami, sausage, or pastrami. It's easy to find deli meats that are almost fat free. Don't use the amount of meat often given on many deli-made sandwiches. An appropriate portion is 2 slices, or around 2 ounces. Some delis serve 4 to 8 ounces! If you are a fan of salami, the Cold-Cut Combo recipe (page 116) will show you how you can fit some higher-fat options into your *Volumetrics Eating Plan*.
- Mayonnaise-based fillings such as tuna, chicken, or egg salad can be the highest in calories. These are sneaky calories—people often think they are making a healthy choice, not realizing that these sandwiches can easily reach 800 calories. I will show you how to make these popular choices volumetric with the Almond

Chicken Salad Sandwich (page 114), and the Zesty Tuna Salad Pita (page 124). Cutting the mayonnaise saves calories and reduces the energy density, and you can bulk up your sandwich with veggies and even fruit.

- Grilled fresh fish makes a delicious and nutritious filling. Complement it with your favorite vegetables for a satisfying and balanced meal.
- Frozen veggie burgers come in a wide variety of flavors. They are low-calorie and quick to cook, so these can be a good choice when you are in a hurry.
- What you choose to spread on your sandwich to add flavor and moisture can have a big impact on the calorie content. Don't add any fat that you can live without. Butter and other fatty spreads are not necessary for a tasty sandwich. If you can't do without, cut back on the amount you use.
- Substitute reduced-fat versions of your favorite spread. Many people don't notice when reduced-fat mayonnaise, cream cheese, or peanut butter is substituted.
- Make your own reduced-fat spread—try the House Dressing (page 76).
- Hummus is a delicious addition to many types of sandwiches, especially those that combine a variety of vegetables. Try Mel's Fresh Lemon Hummus (page 77), or buy it ready made.
- Add flavor by using strong tasting vegetables such as onions and bell peppers, or try hot peppers, relishes, horseradish, or pickles. Use spicy mustard instead of mayonnaise. Add a few capers or sliced olives. These additions mask reductions in fat content and add variety.
- Fresh herbs can change an ordinary sandwich into one that is much more exotic. Cilantro can take you south of the border, or add basil to fresh mozzarella and tomato for the flavors of Italy.

Try the *Volumetrics* recipes for sandwiches and wraps—then get creative and combine your favorite low-calorie ingredients. Taking time to make a sandwich in the morning can keep you away from the high-energy-dense foods that you will find when shopping for a quick lunch. Follow your sandwich with fruit, such as an apple or a clementine, and you will have a nutritious meal that should keep hunger in check until dinner. Be like me and become a kid again. I take my small personal cooler or lunch box with me to work. In addition to your sandwich, you can load it with low-energy-dense snacks, such as carrot or celery sticks or some low-fat yogurt, and you will be better able to resist the plates of goodies around the office.

Almond Chicken Salad Sandwich

This savory sandwich filling features the delicious combination of grapes and chicken. You can also serve the chicken salad alone on a bed of lettuce without the bread.

1½ cups diced, cooked chicken breast, about 1½ 5-ounce skinless, boneless chicken breast halves (see Cook's Note)
1 cup halved, seedless red grapes
¼ cup diced celery
¼ cup reduced-fat mayonnaise

1 tablespoon toasted slivered almonds (page 84)
½ teaspoon freshly ground pepper
8 thin slices multigrain bread
2 cups shredded green-leaf lettuce

1. Combine the chicken, grapes, celery, mayonnaise, almonds, and pepper together in a medium bowl and mix salad well.

2. Divide the chicken salad evenly on 4 slices of the bread. Top each with ½ cup lettuce and another slice of bread.

YIELD: 4 servings

COOK'S NOTE: If you do not have cooked chicken breast meat, try this easy method. Arrange skinless, boneless chicken breasts in a saucepan. Add enough cold water to cover the chicken. Bring the water to a simmer over low heat. Turn the chicken over, cover, and remove the pan from the heat. Let the chicken sit in the pan for 15 to 20 minutes, or until it is no longer pink in the center. Remove the chicken and refrigerate until ready to use.

Nutritional Information Per Serving

Calories 275 | Energy Density 1.4 | Carbohydrate 35 g. | Fat 6 g. | Protein 18 g. | Fiber 2 g.

Nutritional Information Per Serving of Chicken Salad

Calories 150 | Energy Density 1.4 | Carbohydrate 10 g. | Fat 6 g. | Protein 13 g. | Fiber 1 g.

For a 275-calorie sandwich

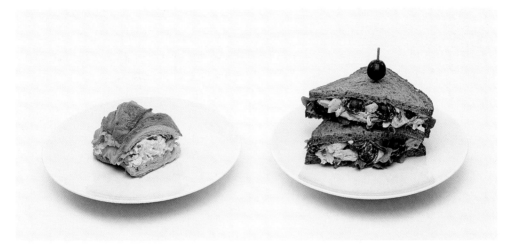

TRADITIONAL	How we lowered the ED	VOLUMETRICS
Chicken salad croissant	▸ Used whole-wheat bread and reduced-fat mayonnaise ▸ Added grapes	Almond Chicken Salad Sandwich

Cold-Cut Combo Sandwich

When you are craving an Italian submarine or hero, try this recipe.

4 tablespoons Italian Dressing (page 153)
2 teaspoons grated Parmesan cheese
1 teaspoon dried oregano or dry Italian
  seasoning
4 split 2-ounce wheat rolls
6 ounces cooked, thinly sliced deli turkey
  breast, about 8 slices
4 ounces capocollo ham, 8 slices

2 ounces reduced-fat Genoa salami,
  4 slices
2 tomatoes, cored and sliced
1 green bell pepper, seeded, sliced into
  rings
¼ cup sliced black olives
1 cup shredded romaine lettuce

1. Combine the dressing, Parmesan, and oregano in a small bowl. Spread the dressing mixture evenly on the bottom of each roll.

2. Divide the turkey among the rolls and top with 2 slices of ham and 1 slice of salami.

3. Divide the tomato slices, pepper rings, olives, and romaine evenly over the 4 sandwiches. Cover each with the top half of a roll.

YIELD: 4 servings

COOK'S NOTE: If you do not like spicy ham, try a milder low-fat ham in place of the capocollo ham.

Nutritional Information Per Serving

Calories 345 | Energy Density 1.2 | Carbohydrate 36 g. | Fat 10 g. | Protein 27 g. | Fiber 4 g.

Mediterranean Turkey Sandwich

The varied textures and flavors from the sun-dried tomatoes, avocado, and red peppers add interest to this sandwich.

3 tablespoons nonfat mayonnaise
1 tablespoon sun-dried tomato paste
8 thin slices multigrain bread
6 ounces oven-roasted or smoked sliced
   deli turkey breast, about 8 slices

½ avocado, peeled and pitted
½ large cucumber, unpeeled
½ cup roasted red bell pepper strips
1 cup baby spinach

1. Stir the mayonnaise and tomato paste together.

2. Spread 1 tablespoon of the mayonnaise mixture on each of 4 slices of the bread. Divide the turkey among the bread slices.

3. Cut the avocado and cucumber into 8 slices each. Top the turkey with 2 slices of avocado and cucumber.

4. Divide the pepper strips among the 4 sandwiches. Top each with ¼ cup spinach and a slice of multigrain bread.

YIELD: 4 servings

Nutritional Information Per Serving

Calories 300 | Energy Density 1.4 | Carbohydrate 41 g. | Fat 7 g. | Protein 19 g. | Fiber 7 g.

Open-Faced Roast Beef Sandwich

Using only one slice of rye bread and adding lots of peppers and onions, lowered the energy density of this sandwich. Pictured on page 56.

1½ cups sliced bell peppers, any
   combination of red, yellow, and/or green
1 cup sliced mushrooms, about 2½ ounces
¾ cup sliced red onions
2 tablespoons reduced-fat mayonnaise
2 teaspoons prepared horseradish, drained,
   or to taste

4 thin slices rye bread
8 ounces thinly sliced, lean, deli roast beef,
   about 10 slices
4 tablespoons shredded Swiss cheese

1. Preheat the broiler.

2. In a nonstick skillet coated with cooking spray, sauté the peppers, mushrooms, and onions over medium heat for 5 minutes, or until slightly tender.

3. Combine the mayonnaise and horseradish and spread evenly over the rye slices.

4. Divide the roast beef among the slices of bread.

5. Divide the sautéed vegetables evenly over the sandwiches and top each with 1 tablespoon cheese.

6. Place the sandwiches on a baking sheet and broil until the cheese melts.

YIELD: 4 servings.

COOK'S NOTE: Chicken or turkey breast can be substituted for the roast beef; omit the horseradish.

Nutritional Information Per Serving

Calories 200 | Energy Density 1.1 | Carbohydrate 19 g. | Fat 8 g. | Protein 15 g. | Fiber 2 g.

Roasted Portobello Sandwich

With their substantial texture and flavor, portobello mushrooms provide a satisfying alternative to meat. Have this flavorful, vegetable-packed sandwich as the main part of your lunch or dinner.

½ cup lime juice

2 tablespoons extra-virgin olive oil

½ cup red-wine vinegar

1 tablespoon minced garlic

2 teaspoons chopped fresh cilantro

2 teaspoons sugar

½ teaspoon salt

¼ teaspoon freshly ground black pepper

4 large cleaned portobello mushroom caps, about 4 inches in diameter

8 teaspoons Guacamole (page 88)

4 split onion Kaiser rolls

½ cup baby spinach

½ cup sliced roasted red bell peppers

½ cup scrubbed, unpeeled sliced cucumber

4 slices tomatoes

4 slices reduced-fat pepper-Jack cheese

1. In a small bowl, combine ½ cup water, lime juice, oil, vinegar, garlic, cilantro, sugar, salt, and pepper. Place the mixture, along with the mushroom caps, in a resealable plastic bag and marinate 1 hour.

2. Preheat the oven to 400 degrees.

3. Remove the mushroom caps from the marinade and place on a baking sheet, stem side up. Roast for 15 minutes, or until brown and tender.

4. Spread 1 teaspoon of guacamole on each half of the Kaiser rolls. Divide the spinach, red bell peppers, and cucumber over the guacamole. Top each with a tomato slice, a mushroom cap, a cheese slice, and the top half of each roll.

YIELD: 4 servings

COOK'S NOTE: To pack this as part of your lunch, don't add the cooked mushrooms to the sandwich until you are ready to eat.

Nutritional Information Per Serving

Calories 290 | Energy Density 1.2 | Carbohydrate 40 g. | Fat 10 g. | Protein 11 g. | Fiber 4 g.

Buffalo Chicken Wraps

Try these wraps instead of fried chicken wings. The baked chicken paired with hot-pepper sauce and a low-fat blue cheese dressing gives you that comfort-food taste.

2 cups shredded, cooked chicken breast meat (page 114)
2 tablespoons hot-pepper sauce
½ cup reduced-fat blue cheese dressing
4 10" wheat tortillas

2 cups shredded romaine lettuce
1 cup diced celery
1 cup peeled, seeded, and diced cucumber
1 cup peeled, shredded carrots

1. Combine the chicken and hot-pepper sauce in a small bowl.

2. Spread 2 tablespoons of blue cheese dressing over each tortilla. Arrange ½ cup romaine horizontally down the center of each tortilla. Top each with ½ cup chicken, ¼ cup celery, ¼ cup cucumber, and ¼ cup carrots.

3. Fold the sides of each tortilla toward the center. Starting from the bottom, tightly roll the tortilla up to the top.

YIELD: 4 servings

COOK'S NOTE: Try using flavored tortillas to add color and extra flavor.

Nutritional Information Per Serving

Calories 350 | Energy Density 1.2 | Carbohydrate 45 g. | Fat 7 g. | Protein 28 g. | Fiber 4 g.

For a 350-calorie wrap

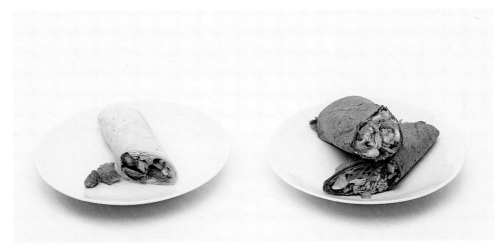

TRADITIONAL	How we lowered the ED	VOLUMETRICS
Fried chicken wrap	▸ Used baked chicken instead of fried ▸ Used reduced-fat blue cheese dressing ▸ Added more veggies	Buffalo Chicken Wrap

Asian Chicken Wraps

In this quick-to-prepare wrap, traditional mu shu pancakes are replaced by flour tortillas.

2 tablespoons hoisin sauce

1 tablespoon vegetable oil

2 cups shredded Chinese or Napa cabbage

2 cups bean sprouts

4 cups sliced mushrooms, about 11 ounces

1 cup diced, cooked chicken breast
   (page 114)

4 flour tortillas

1. In a small bowl, combine the hoisin sauce and 1 tablespoon water, and set it aside.

2. Heat the oil over medium heat in a large skillet coated with cooking spray. Add the cabbage, bean sprouts, and mushrooms and stir-fry 5 to 7 minutes, or until tender.

3. Stir in the chicken and hoisin sauce mixture and cook 1 to 2 minutes, or until thoroughly heated. Divide among the tortillas.

4. Fold the sides of each tortilla toward the center. Starting from the bottom, tightly roll the tortilla up to the top.

YIELD: 4 servings

Nutritional Information Per Serving

Calories 310 | Energy Density 1.1 | Carbohydrate 29 g. | Fat 9 g. | Protein 29 g. | Fiber 4 g.

Chicken and Avocado Pita Pockets

For a new twist on your packed lunch, fill whole-wheat pita pockets with veggies and low-fat chicken breast for added satiety.

1 pound cooked chicken breast, cut into
  ½-inch pieces (page 114)
¼ cup shredded reduced-fat Cheddar
  cheese
¾ cup diced avocado
½ cup seeded, chopped bell peppers, any
  color
½ cup chopped celery

½ cup unpeeled chopped cucumber
½ cup peeled, shredded carrots
½ cup finely chopped cauliflowerettes
¼ cup chopped red onions
1 cup Balsamic Dressing (page 152)
4 6" whole-wheat pitas, cut in half
  crosswise

1. Toss the chicken, Cheddar, and vegetables with the dressing. Fill each pita half with approximately ¾ cup of the chicken mixture.

YIELD: 4 servings of 2 halves

Nutritional Information Per Serving

Calories 375 | Energy density 1.3 | Carbohydrate 47 g. | Fat 10 g. | Protein 27 g. | Fiber 8 g.

Zesty Tuna Salad Pita

Dijon mustard sparks the flavor of this salad, and the vegetables add crunch.

2 tablespoons Dijon mustard
2 tablespoons reduced-fat mayonnaise
½ cup chopped red onions
½ cup seeded, chopped red bell peppers
½ cup seeded, chopped yellow bell peppers
½ cup chopped celery

1 12-ounce can solid white tuna packed in
   water, drained and flaked
Pinch freshly ground black pepper
4 6-inch whole-wheat pita pockets
½ cup shredded arugula or spinach
½ cup sliced mushrooms, about 1⅓ ounces

For a 285-calorie pita

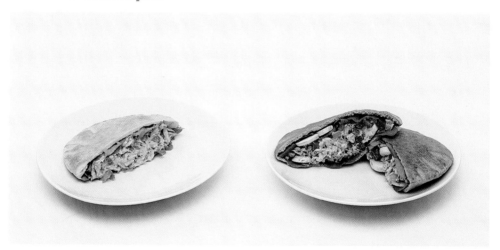

TRADITIONAL	How we lowered the ED	VOLUMETRICS
Tuna salad pita	▸ Used tuna packed in water and reduced-fat mayo ▸ Added more vegetables	Zesty Tuna Salad Pita

1. Whisk the mustard and mayonnaise in a medium bowl.

2. Add the onions, bell peppers, celery, tuna, and black pepper. Stir the tuna salad until well mixed; set aside.

3. Cut the pitas in half crosswise.

4. Divide the arugula, mushrooms, and tuna salad among the pita halves.

YIELD: 4 servings

COOK'S NOTE: You can combine the arugula, mushrooms, and tuna mixture and serve it on a bed of lettuce or on whole-wheat bread.

Nutritional Information Per Serving

Calories 285 | Energy Density 1.2 | Carbohydrate 32 g. | Fat 6 g. | Protein 27 g. | Fiber 6 g.

Nutritional Information Per Serving of Tuna Salad

Calories 155 | Energy Density 0.90 | Carbohydrate 6 g. | Fat 5 g. | Protein 21 g. | Fiber 1 g.

All American Hamburger

By using low-fat ground beef, it is possible to have a great tasting burger. Seasonings and condiments give the meat flavor and keep it moist.

1 pound 95 percent lean ground beef

⅓ cup chopped onions

2 tablespoons ketchup

2 tablespoons Worcestershire sauce

1 teaspoon hot-pepper sauce

6 split, 2-ounce, wheat rolls

1½ cups shredded romaine lettuce

2 tomatoes, cored and sliced

½ cup sliced red onions

1. Combine the beef, onions, ketchup, Worcestershire sauce, and hot-pepper sauce. Form into 6 equal sized burger patties.

2. Cook the burgers in a large, nonstick skillet sprayed with cooking spray over medium to medium-high heat until no longer pink, approximately 8 to 10 minutes.

3. Place one burger on the bottom half of each roll. Divide the romaine, tomatoes, and onions evenly over each burger and cover with the roll top.

YIELD: 6 servings

Nutritional Information Per Serving

Calories 310 | Energy Density 1.5 | Carbohydrate 34 g. | Fat 7 g. | Protein 28 g. | Fiber 3 g.

7 Salads and Salad Dressings

Salad can lull you into thinking you are eating a low-calorie meal. Even though lettuce and other vegetables don't have a lot of calories, much of the fat and the calories many of us eat in a day come from salad dressing.

SALAD AND SATIETY: HOW HAVING SALAD FIRST CAN HELP YOU TO EAT LESS

In 2003, at the annual meeting of the North American Association for the Study of Obesity, I presented a new study "Salad and Satiety." To my amazement, the study was featured in the *Wall Street Journal,* the *Washington Post,* and *USA Today,* as well as on ABC's *World News Tonight.* Why was salad such big news? Because we showed for the first time that eating salad as a first course could subtract calories from a meal. The answer for calorie reduction was to eat more, not less! Beginning a meal with a large portion of a low-energy-dense garden salad is an effective strategy for reducing how many calories you eat during a meal if the salad is big in volume and low in calories.

In our study, people ate fewer calories of a second course of pasta when their meal started with 3 cups of low-energy-dense salad (100 calories) compared to when they didn't have a salad. Although they ate 100 calories less at lunch when the salad was included, they didn't feel any hungrier. Eating a smaller portion of the salad (1½ cups instead of 3 cups) also reduced the number of calories eaten at lunch, just not as much as the bigger portion. Bigger can be better for weight management if you do it right by keeping the energy density low!

You are probably wondering how we reduced the energy density of the salad and how it tasted. The answer is in the dressings and toppings—we used nonfat Italian dressing and reduced-fat cheese. And according to taste ratings given by the study participants, the salad tasted good. This salad worked so well as a way to reduce calories that I am going to give you the recipe for the Volumetrics Salad (page 134). If you don't like using nonfat or reduced-fat products, you will need to experiment to see how little oil (or dressing) you need to make your salad tasty. To help you, we have included some of our favorite *Volumetrics* salad dressings (pages 152–153). Fat helps your body absorb nutrients from vegetables, so if you are having just salad, don't eliminate all of the fat.

MAIN-COURSE SALADS

Sticking to salads made primarily of vegetables is the easiest way to ensure you are eating a satisfying amount that will fill you up, but all kinds of salads can be volumetric and fit in your menu plan. For example, we have shown that lowering the energy density of a pasta salad provides satisfaction with fewer calories. In one study, we lowered the energy density of a main-course salad by adding more vegetables and using less pasta. The people in the study liked the new, lower-energy-dense version as much as the original pasta salad. Even though they could eat as much as they liked, they ended up eating the same weight of the lower-energy-dense salad and about 30 percent fewer calories than that of the higher-energy-dense salad. To show you how easy it is to reduce the energy density of a main-course salad, we have included the recipe for the tasty lower-energy-dense pasta salad from this study, Liz's Pasta Salad (page 146).

Your best options for main-course salads are similar to those for side salads, but they should be bigger and higher in calories. You should keep the proportion of veggies high, and keep the fat down by carefully selecting the type of dressing and reducing the amount of dressing, cheese, and croutons. To boost satiety, add lean protein such as grilled chicken breast, chickpeas, or red beans. Try the California Cobb Salad (page 143) or the Santa Fe Steak Salad (page 144) to see how satisfying salad can be.

Here are some tips to make sure you choose your salads wisely.

- The bigger the better, so long as it is low in energy density and packed with your favorite vegetables.
- Add an extra cup of lettuce or other vegetables to your usual tossed salad without increasing the amount of salad dressing. Choose flavorful veggies such as red or yellow bell peppers, ripe tomatoes, or onions and you won't miss the dressing.
- Add fruit to reduce the energy density—sliced fresh pears, strawberries, grapes, orange sections, or canned mandarin oranges are great for adding flavor. The Fresh Fruit and Spinach Salad recipe (page 138) is delicious.
- Use only as many high-fat additions such as dressing, cheese, and croutons as you need to enjoy the dish.
- Don't want to give up the oil? Use less oil, but choose one that has lots of flavor such as extra-virgin olive, walnut, or sesame oil.
- Bump up the proportion of lemon juice or vinegar in your dressing.
- Experiment with fat-free flavorings such as mustard, Worcestershire sauce, fresh herbs, citrus zest, or minced garlic.
- Instead of topping your salad with lots of high-fat cheese, try:
  - A sprinkle of high-flavor cheese such as Parmesan
  - Low-fat or nonfat cheese mixed in with the regular cheese: People in our studies didn't notice the difference
  - Reduced-fat cottage cheese
- It is okay to use small amounts of avocado, nuts, or olives as toppings—although these toppings are higher in energy density, they contain healthy fats.
- Try using a variety of lettuces: Boston, red leaf, green leaf, arugula, romaine, radicchio—they will add interesting flavors, textures, and colors.
- Add lean protein such as grilled chicken breast, chickpeas, lentils, or white beans for added satiety, especially if the salad is your main course.
- In a restaurant, order dressing on the side, then be careful about how much you use!
- At a buffet, fill your plate with low-energy-dense salads to crowd out the high-energy-dense options.
- If salad is your usual fast-food choice, make sure you know what you are eating. Most fast-food chains provide nutrition information online, and some provide it at the restaurants.

Charlie's Greek Salad

This is a rustic side salad based on one Charlie was served during a trip to Athens. The feta cheese, although not in the original, adds another layer of flavor.

½ teaspoon salt

Freshly ground black pepper

1 tablespoon fresh lemon juice

1 tablespoon extra-virgin olive oil

2 cups scrubbed, unpeeled, and unseeded cucumber, quartered lengthwise, and

cut crosswise into ½-inch pieces, about ½ pound

2 cups cored tomatoes cut into ½-inch cubes

¼ cup chopped fresh oregano

¼ cup crumbled, nonfat feta cheese

1. Whisk the salt, several grindings of pepper, lemon juice, and oil in a large bowl. Add the cucumber, tomatoes, oregano, and feta. Toss gently, but well.

YIELD: 4 servings of ¾ cup each

COOK'S NOTE: This dish is best when tomatoes and cucumbers are at their peak.

Nutritional Information Per Serving

Calories 80 | Energy Density 0.50 | Carbohydrate 6 g. | Fat 6 g. | Protein 2 g. | Fiber 1 g.

For an 80-calorie salad

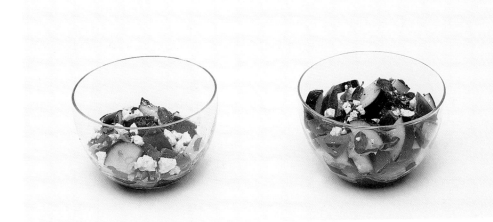

TRADITIONAL	How we lowered the ED	VOLUMETRICS
Greek salad	▸ Reduced oil ▸ Substituted nonfat feta cheese ▸ Omitted cured olives ▸ Increased the veggies	Charlie's Greek Salad

Creamy Cucumber and Dill Salad

This light, refreshing side dish goes well with fish and seafood. Pictured on page 4.

4 cups thinly sliced seedless cucumber,
    about 1 pound
1 teaspoon salt
⅓ cup Yogurt Cheese (page 89)

2 tablespoons rice-wine vinegar
2 tablespoons minced fresh dill
Pinch freshly ground black pepper
1 cup thinly sliced red onions

1. Toss the cucumber and ½ teaspoon salt in a colander set over a larger bowl. Let stand for 30 minutes, stirring occasionally. Rinse and dry the cucumber slices. Discard the liquid.

2. Whisk the yogurt cheese, vinegar, ½ teaspoon salt, dill, and pepper in a large bowl until smooth.

3. Add the cucumber and onions and toss to coat.

4. Cover the bowl and chill the salad, 1 hour.

YIELD: 4 servings of ¾ cup each

COOK'S NOTE: Add ½ cup thinly sliced red radishes to the salad to give it some color and a sharper taste.

Nutritional Information Per Serving

Calories 50 | Energy Density 0.28 | Carbohydrate 9 g. | Fat 1 g. | Protein 3 g. | Fiber 1 g.

Fennel, Orange, and Arugula Salad

Oranges, along with the distinctive taste of arugula and the crunchy texture of the fennel, make this a bright and refreshing side salad.

2 large navel oranges
1 tablespoon orange juice
1 tablespoon extra-virgin olive oil
¼ teaspoon salt

Pinch freshly ground black pepper
1 fennel bulb, about 1¼ pounds
4 cups shredded arugula

1. Grate 2 teaspoons orange zest. Peel the oranges, making sure to remove all the bitter white pith. Cut the flesh into ½" thick slices and cut the slices crosswise into cubes.

2. Whisk the zest, orange juice, oil, salt, and pepper in a large bowl.

3. Remove the fennel stalks and chop enough of the fronds to measure 1 tablespoon. Cut the bulb lengthwise into quarters. Cut out and discard the core. Cut each quarter crosswise into thin slices.

4. Toss the orange cubes, fennel, fennel fronds, and arugula with the dressing.

YIELD: 4 servings of 1 cup each

Nutritional Information Per Serving

Calories 80 | Energy Density 0.58 | Carbohydrate 13 g. | Fat 4 g. | Protein 2 g. | Fiber 4 g.

Volumetrics Salad

This is the salad used in one of the research studies at my lab. Serve this salad as a first course and it will fill you up so that you eat less during the rest of the meal.

8 cups mixed salad greens

1 cup peeled, shredded carrots

1 cup diced celery

1 cup cored, diced tomatoes

1 cup scrubbed, unpeeled diced cucumber

6 tablespoons shredded nonfat mozzarella cheese

¾ cup Italian Dressing (page 153)

1. Mix all the vegetables in a large bowl.

2. Add the mozzarella and Italian Dressing and toss well.

3. Divide the mixture among 4 salad bowls or plates.

YIELD: 4 servings of 3 cups each

COOK'S NOTE: This recipe uses the low-fat Italian Dressing (page 153) rather than a nonfat Italian dressing as noted in the introduction to this chapter. If you prefer a nonfat dressing, try one of the commercially available nonfat Italian dressings.

Nutritional Information Per Serving

Calories 100 | Energy Density 0.30 | Carbohydrate 16 g. | Fat 2 g. | Protein 5 g. | Fiber 4 g.

For a 100-calorie salad

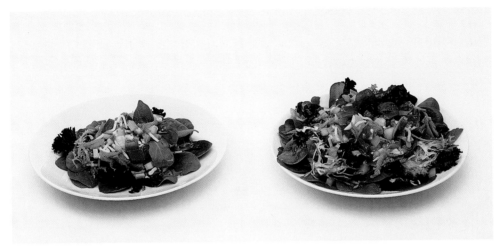

TRADITIONAL	How we lowered the ED	VOLUMETRICS
Tossed salad	► Used low-fat Italian dressing and reduced-fat cheese ► Added more vegetables	Volumetrics Salad

Lemony Fennel Salad

Fresh fennel has a mild licorice taste that is balanced nicely by the lemon. This attractive side salad makes a tasty addition to a picnic basket. The energy density is so low that you can enjoy a large satisfying portion.

½ teaspoon lemon zest

2 tablespoons lemon juice

2 teaspoons extra-virgin olive oil

¼ teaspoon salt

1 fennel bulb, about 1¼ pounds

1½ teaspoons grated Parmesan cheese

1. Whisk the lemon zest, lemon juice, oil, salt, and 1 tablespoon water in a large bowl.

2. Remove the fennel stalks and finely chop enough of the fronds to measure 2 tablespoons and add to the bowl of dressing. Cut the bulbs in quarters lengthwise. Cut out and discard the core. Cut each quarter crosswise into thin slices.

3. Add the fennel slices to the bowl and toss well. Sprinkle with Parmesan and toss again.

YIELD: 4 servings of ½ cup each

Nutritional Information Per Serving

Calories 55 | Energy Density 0.36 | Carbohydrate 8 g. | Fat 2 g. | Protein 1 g. | Fiber 3 g.

Insalata Mista

Radicchio adds a vivid red accent and a peppery flavor to this side salad.

1 fennel bulb, about 1¼ pounds
4 cups torn Boston lettuce
3 cups torn radicchio
1 tablespoon extra-virgin olive oil

¼ teaspoon salt
Pinch freshly ground black pepper
3 to 4 tablespoons freshly squeezed
  lemon juice

1. Remove the fennel stalks and finely chop enough of the fronds to measure 2 tablespoons. Cut the bulbs in quarters lengthwise. Cut out and discard the core. Cut each quarter crosswise into thin slices.

2. In a large bowl, toss the fennel, fennel fronds, Boston lettuce, and radicchio with the oil, salt, and pepper. Add 3 tablespoons lemon juice and toss again. Taste and add more lemon juice, if desired.

3. Divide the salad among 4 salad plates or bowls.

YIELD: 4 servings of 1¾ cups each

Nutritional Information Per Serving

Calories 60 | Energy Density 0.39 | Carbohydrate 7g. | Fat 4 g. | Protein 1 g. | Fiber 3 g.

Fresh Fruit and Spinach Salad with Orange–Poppy Seed Dressing

This salad is a favorite in my lab when we have a party. It is a sweet way to eat your spinach.

½ cup low-fat plain yogurt
¼ cup nonfat milk
¼ cup sugar
2 tablespoons distilled white vinegar
2 tablespoons orange juice
1 tablespoon poppy seeds
1 cup sliced fresh strawberries

1 orange, peeled and segmented
½ cup fresh blueberries
½ cup diced fresh pineapple
1 tablespoon toasted almond slices
  (page 84)
8 cups baby spinach

1. Place the yogurt, milk, sugar, vinegar, juice, and poppy seeds in a screw-top jar. Shake vigorously until blended. Set the Orange-Poppy Seed Dressing aside.

2. Combine the fruit and toasted almonds in a medium bowl and mix well.

3. Divide the baby spinach evenly among 4 salad plates or bowls. Top each with ¼ fruit mixture (a little over ½ cup each).

4. Spoon 2 tablespoons of the Orange–Poppy Seed Dressing over each salad.

YIELD: 4 servings of 2½ cups each

COOK'S NOTE: Canned pineapple and mandarin oranges may be used in place of fresh fruit.

Nutritional Information Per Serving

Calories 150 | Energy Density 0.64 | Carbohydrate 30 g. | Fat 2 g. | Protein 4 g. | Fiber 8 g.

Nutritional Information Per Serving of Dressing

Calories 45 | Energy Density 1.2 | Carbohydrate 8 g. | Fat 1 g. | Protein 1 g. | Fiber 0 g.

Tangy Cole Slaw

Reminiscent of my mother's cole slaw, this side salad has the tangy flavor of dill pickle.

⅓ cup reduced-fat mayonnaise

1 cup diced dill pickle

3 tablespoons dill-pickle juice

1 teaspoon celery seed

3½ cups shredded green cabbage, about 1 pound

½ cup peeled, shredded carrots

½ cup diced celery

1. Whisk the mayonnaise, pickle, pickle juice, and celery seed in a large bowl.

2. Add the cabbage, carrots, and celery to the bowl and toss well. Chill 1 hour before serving.

YIELD: 4 servings of 1 cup each

COOK'S NOTE: This salad is best if eaten on the same day it is prepared. Bagged, shredded cole slaw mix can be used in place of the cabbage and carrots to shorten preparation time.

Nutritional Information Per Serving

Calories 65 | Energy Density 0.43 | Carbohydrate 12 g. | Fat 2 g. | Protein 2 g. | Fiber 3 g.

Pepper Slaw

This light and tart salad makes a colorful side dish.

2¾ cups shredded green cabbage

1 cup shredded purple cabbage

½ cup seeded, diced green bell peppers

¼ cup peeled, shredded carrots

2 tablespoons sugar

¼ cup cider vinegar

½ tablespoon vegetable oil

½ teaspoon freshly ground black pepper

1. Combine the cabbage, peppers, and carrots in a large bowl.

2. In a separate bowl, whisk the sugar, vinegar, oil, and black pepper.

3. Pour the dressing over the cabbage and toss well. Refrigerate 2 hours before serving.

YIELD: 4 servings of ¾ cup each

COOK'S NOTE: To reduce preparation time, 3 cups of prepared, shredded cole slaw mix can be used in place of the green cabbage and carrots. This dish is best if served on the same day it is prepared.

Nutritional Information Per Serving

Calories 65 | Energy Density 0.60 | Carbohydrate 12 g. | Fat 2 g. | Protein 1 g. | Fiber 2 g.

For a 65-calorie side dish

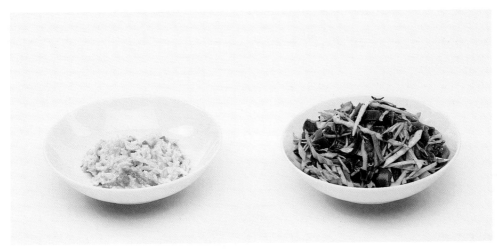

TRADITIONAL	How we lowered the ED	VOLUMETRICS
Cole slaw	▶ Used vinegar and a small amount of sugar in place of mayonnaise	Pepper Slaw

Thai Chicken Salad

Peanuts and peanut oil give this refreshing main dish salad a distinctive Thai taste.

½ cup sliced scallions

1 tablespoon minced garlic

1 seeded and minced jalapeno

3 tablespoons lime juice

3 tablespoons reduced-sodium soy sauce

2 tablespoons honey

1 tablespoon peanut oil

1 tablespoon rice-wine vinegar or distilled
   white vinegar

7 cups torn romaine lettuce

1 cup shredded red cabbage

1 cup peeled, grated carrots

1 cup seeded, diced red bell peppers

1 cup peeled, seeded, chopped cucumber

1 cup small snow-pea pods

2 cups cooked, diced chicken breast
   (page 114)

4 teaspoons crushed unsalted, dry-roasted
   peanuts

1. Whisk the scallions, garlic, jalapeno, juice, soy sauce, honey, peanut oil, vinegar, and 2 tablespoons water in a large bowl. Set aside for 30 minutes.

2. Whisk the dressing to recombine and add the lettuce, cabbage, carrots, bell peppers, cucumber, and pea pods to the bowl. Toss well.

3. Divide the salad among 4 plates. Top each with the chicken and peanuts.

YIELD: 4 servings of 3 cups each

COOK'S NOTE: For a more authentic Thai flavor, substitute 3 tablespoons fish sauce for the soy sauce.

Nutritional Information Per Serving

Calories 255 | Energy Density 0.71 | Carbohydrate 22 g. | Fat 8 g. | Protein 26 g. | Fiber 5 g.

California Cobb Salad with Nonfat Tomato and Herb Dressing

This popular, visually appealing, main dish gives you a large portion without a lot of calories.

8 cups mixed spring salad greens

2 cups cooked, diced chicken breast meat (page 114)

2 cups halved cherry tomatoes

1 cup chopped cucumber, unpeeled and scrubbed

4 slices cooked turkey bacon, chopped

2 peeled hard boiled eggs, chopped

¾ cup chopped avocado

2 tablespoons chopped fresh chives

4 tablespoons crumbled blue cheese

⅓ cup reduced-sodium vegetable juice

2 tablespoons lemon juice

1 tablespoon chopped, fresh flat-leaf parsley

½ teaspoon chopped garlic

¼ teaspoon salt

Dash dried thyme

Dash sugar

Dash cayenne

Dash freshly ground black pepper

1. Divide the greens among 4 large salad bowls. Divide the chicken, tomato, cucumber, bacon, eggs, and avocado among the salads, arranging each ingredient in an individual row on top of the greens. Sprinkle the chives and blue cheese on top of each salad.

2. Place the rest of the ingredients in a screw-top jar. Shake vigorously until blended and set the Nonfat Tomato and Herb Dressing aside.

3. Serve the salad with the dressing on the side.

YIELD: 4 servings of 3½ cups each

COOK'S NOTE: You can turn this salad into a vegetarian dish by omitting the chicken and the bacon.

Nutritional Information Per Serving

Calories 280 | Energy Density 0.82 | Carbohydrate 12 g. | Fat 13 g. | Protein 31 g. | Fiber 5 g.

Nutritional Information Per 2 Tablespoon Serving of Dressing

Calories 10 | Energy Density 0.27 | Carbohydrate 2 g. | Fat 0 g. | Protein 0 g. | Fiber 0 g.

Santa Fe Steak Salad with Lime-Cilantro Dressing

You can eat steak when following *Volumetrics*, just watch your portion, and combine it with lots of veggies to reduce the energy density. Serve this main dish salad for lunch or dinner.

½ cup lime juice

3 tablespoons extra-virgin olive oil

½ cup chopped fresh cilantro

1 tablespoon chopped garlic

2 teaspoons sugar

1 teaspoon cumin

⅛ teaspoon cayenne

1 pound flank steak, cut diagonally against the grain into ¼-inch thick pieces

8 cups mixed salad greens

1 cup peeled, diced jicama

1 seeded red or green bell pepper, sliced

½ cup chopped red onions

¼ cup chopped green olives

1 cup halved cherry tomatoes

½ cup canned dark-red kidney beans, rinsed and drained

½ cup canned corn, drained

¾ cup diced avocado

½ cup shredded, reduced-fat Mexican-blend cheese

1 cup prepared tomato salsa

1. Combine the lime juice, oil, cilantro, garlic, sugar, cumin, cayenne, and ½ cup of water in a blender. Blend on high until smooth. Set the Lime-Cilantro Dressing aside.

2. Marinate the steak in the dressing for 1 hour.

3. Place a large skillet coated with cooking spray over medium-high heat. When it is hot, add the meat and marinade, and cook, stirring, 3 to 4 minutes, or until the meat is no longer pink. Transfer the meat to a plate and cover.

4. Divide the greens among 4 plates.

5. Mix the jicama, bell peppers, onions, olives, tomatoes, beans, corn, and avocado in a bowl.

6. Divide the jicama mixture among the plates and top with the cheese, salsa, and steak.

YIELD: 4 servings of 3½ cups each

COOK'S NOTE: Jicama, also known as *Mexican potato,* can be found in the produce section of large supermarkets and specialty grocery stores. It is a crunchy tuber that adds wonderful flavor and texture to salads. (When used as a dressing for salad, Lime-Cilantro Dressing yields 12 servings of 1½ tablespoons each.)

Nutritional Information Per Serving

Calories 400 | Energy Density 0.79 | Carbohydrate 29 g. | Fat 18 g. | Protein 33 g. | Fiber 10 g.

Nutritional Information Per 1½ Tablespoon Serving of Dressing

Calories 40 | Energy Density 1.6 | Carbohydrate 2 g. | Fat 4 g. | Protein 0 g. | Fiber 0 g.

Liz's Pasta Salad

Liz Bell, one of my doctoral students, developed this main-course pasta salad for use in one of our studies. The participants in the study enjoyed this tasty salad and ate fewer calories than when served a traditional pasta salad.

4 cups ditalini or small shell pasta, cooked and drained

2 cups peeled, shredded carrots

2 cups cored, diced tomatoes

2 cups diced zucchini

2 cups frozen baby peas, cooked and drained

8 tablespoons ¼-inch thick diced ham, about 4 ounces

1 cup shredded part-skim mozzarella cheese

½ cup Italian Dressing (page 153)

1. Combine all the ingredients in a medium bowl and mix well, evenly distributing the dressing. Serve chilled or at room temperature on 4 plates.

YIELD: 4 servings of 3 cups each

COOK'S NOTE: You can use whole-wheat pasta in this recipe for extra fiber.

Nutritional Information Per Serving

Calories 400 | Energy Density 0.80 | Carbohydrate 54 g. | Fat 11 g. | Protein 27 g. | Fiber 9 g.

For a 400-calorie salad

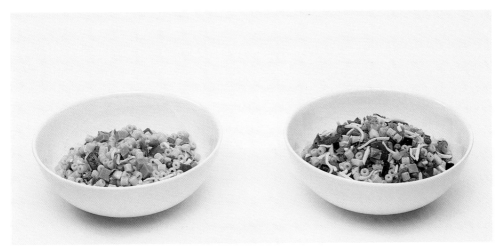

TRADITIONAL	How we lowered the ED	VOLUMETRICS
Pasta salad	▸ Used less pasta ▸ Used a reduced-calorie dressing ▸ Added 4 times the veggies	Liz's Pasta Salad

Tabbouleh

The addition of fennel gives a new twist to this light Lebanese bulgur salad.

⅔ cup bulgur

4 thinly sliced scallions

2 cups chopped, fresh flat-leaf parsley

¼ cup shredded fresh mint

½ cup cored, chopped tomatoes

½ cup chopped celery

½ cup cored, chopped fennel bulb,
   about ¼ bulb

3 tablespoons extra-virgin olive oil

¼ cup lemon juice

¼ teaspoon salt

¼ teaspoon freshly ground black pepper

1. Place the bulgur in a small bowl and cover with water. Let it soak for about 30 minutes.

2. Drain the bulgur through a cheesecloth-lined sieve. Extract as much water as possible by squeezing the cheesecloth. Transfer the bulgur to a medium bowl and fluff with a fork.

3. Combine the scallions, parsley, mint, tomatoes, celery, and fennel with the bulgur.

4. Whisk the oil, lemon juice, salt, and pepper in a small bowl. Pour the dressing over the salad and toss gently to coat. Cover and chill 30 minutes.

YIELD: 8 servings of ½ cup each

Nutritional Information Per Serving

Calories 100 | Energy Density 1.0 | Carbohydrate 13 g. | Fat 6 g. | Protein 2 g. | Fiber 3 g.

Potato Salad with Green Beans and Tarragon

This tangy side dish is delicious served either warm or at room temperature.

4 unpeeled, medium boiling potatoes about
   1 pound, each cut into 8 wedges
½ pound trimmed fresh green beans
1 tablespoon white-wine vinegar
¼ cup chopped scallions

2 tablespoons chopped fresh tarragon
1 tablespoon Dijon mustard
1 tablespoon extra-virgin olive oil
1 teaspoon salt
¼ teaspoon freshly ground black pepper

1. Put the potatoes in a 4- to 5-quart pot and add enough water to cover by 2 inches. Simmer 15 minutes. Add the beans and simmer 7 minutes, or until the potatoes and beans are tender. Drain well.

2. Whisk the rest of the ingredients in a large bowl. Add the potatoes and beans, and toss gently to coat.

YIELD: 4 servings of 1 cup each

COOK'S NOTE: Any white- or red-skinned boiling potato can be used in this recipe.

Nutritional Information Per Serving

Calories 155 | Energy Density 0.80 | Carbohydrate 27 g. | Fat 4 g. | Protein 3 g. | Fiber 4 g.

Tuna and White Bean Salad

Serve this light, flavorful, and slightly tart salad with soup for lunch.

3 tablespoons lemon juice
1 tablespoon extra-virgin olive oil
1 teaspoon minced garlic
1 teaspoon Dijon mustard
½ teaspoon salt
Freshly ground black pepper
1 cup canned cannellini beans,
   rinsed and drained

½ cup chopped red onions
¼ cup pitted, chopped Niçoise olives
2 cups peeled, seeded, and diced tomatoes
3 cups baby spinach
1 12-ounce can solid white tuna,
   packed in water, drained and flaked

1. Whisk the lemon juice, oil, garlic, mustard, salt, several grindings of black pepper, and 2 tablespoons water in a large bowl.

2. Place the rest of the ingredients in the bowl and toss to coat with dressing.

YIELD: 4 servings of 1¾ cups each

COOK'S NOTE: Any white bean can be substituted for the cannellini. Other cured olives such as kalamata can be used in place of the Niçoise.

Nutritional Information Per Serving

Calories 200 | Energy Density 0.66 | Carbohydrate 16 g. | Fat 7 g. | Protein 24 g. | Fiber 6 g.

For a 200-calorie salad

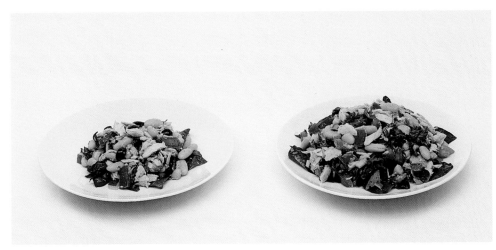

TRADITIONAL	How we lowered the ED	VOLUMETRICS
Salad Niçoise	▸ Decreased oil ▸ Used tuna packed in water ▸ Added more vegetables	Tuna and White Bean Salad

Balsamic Dressing

3 tablespoons balsamic vinegar
1 tablespoon extra-virgin olive oil

¼ teaspoon salt
Pinch freshly ground black pepper

1. Place all the ingredients and 2 tablespoons water in a screw-top jar. Shake vigorously until blended.

YIELD: 4 servings of 1½ tablespoons each

COOK'S NOTE: Aged balsamic vinegar from Modena, Italy has a more intense flavor than domestic varieties. If you use an aged balsamic, you can reduce the amount in this recipe to about 2 tablespoons or less, depending on its intensity.

Nutritional Information Per Serving

Calories 45 | Energy Density 2.0 | Carbohydrate 3 g. | Fat 4 g. | Protein 0 g. | Fiber 0 g.

Dijon Vinaigrette

3 tablespoons white-wine vinegar
1 teaspoon Dijon mustard
1 tablespoon extra-virgin
    olive oil

3 tablespoons nonfat, reduced-sodium
    chicken broth
½ teaspoon salt
Pinch freshly ground black pepper

1. Place all the ingredients in a screw-top jar. Shake vigorously until blended.

YIELD: 4 servings of 2 tablespoons each

Nutritional Information Per Serving

Calories 35 | Energy Density 1.2 | Carbohydrate 0 g. | Fat 4 g. | Protein 0 g. | Fiber 0 g.

Citrus-Ginger Dressing

3 tablespoons lime juice
   from about 1 lime
2 tablespoons extra-virgin olive oil
½ teaspoon sugar

1 tablespoon minced fresh chives
1 teaspoon minced fresh ginger
¼ teaspoon salt
Pinch freshly ground black pepper

1. Place all the ingredients and 2 tablespoons water in a screw-top jar. Shake vigorously until blended.

YIELD: 4 servings of 1½ tablespoons each

Nutritional Information Per Serving.

Calories 65 | Energy Density 3.1 | Carbohydrate 2 g. | Fat 7 g. | Protein 0 g. | Fiber 0 g.

Italian Dressing

3 tablespoons white-wine vinegar
1 tablespoon extra-virgin olive oil

¼ teaspoon salt
Pinch freshly ground black pepper

1. Place all the ingredients and 2 tablespoons water in a screw-top jar. Shake vigorously until blended.

YIELD: 4 servings of 1½ tablespoons each

Nutritional Information Per Serving

Calories 45 | Energy Density 2.0 | Carbohydrate 3 g. | Fat 4 g. | Protein 0 g. | Fiber 0 g.

8 Vegetables and Vegetarian Dishes

Vegetables are key to weight management and good health, and many of us are not eating enough of them. Most vegetables are rich in water and fiber and low in energy density—a satiety-enhancing combination. Studies in my lab have confirmed this high-satiety effect when meals were bulked up with vegetables to reduce the energy density. During a family-style meal, people tend to help themselves to the same amount of food regardless of the energy density. This means that, when the energy density is lowered by adding vegetables, they end up eating *fewer calories!* Equally important, they were just as full and didn't eat more later in the day. In the long term, these saved calories will mean a lower body weight. Studies show that people who were encouraged to eat more vegetables (and I don't mean fries!) and fruit in weight-loss trials lost more weight than those who just cut fat and sugar intake.

Some of you may be saying that this will never work for you—you just don't like many vegetables. Perhaps you were not served many veggies as a child, so you never acquired a taste for them. Don't worry, we have lots of strategies to help you and your family eat more vegetables. An important message for parents is to make sure your own kids get an opportunity to try a wide variety of vegetables. And don't give up if they reject them or don't like them the first few times. Research shows that young children may need to try new foods up to ten times before they really like them.

Back to what you can do if you dislike vegetables. It may be that you are particularly sensitive to bitter compounds in some vegetables such as cabbage or Brussels sprouts. If this is the case, there are some simple strategies you can try to turn this aversion around.

- Add vegetables to dishes such as pastas, stews, and soups.
- Eat younger vegetables, like baby carrots—they are often less bitter. You can find them all year round, both fresh and frozen.
- Add a little butter, oil, or cheese. If adding a small amount of fat means that you will eat your veggies, go for it!
- Some people find adding a sprinkle of sugar to vegetables can cut the bitter taste.

When it comes to vegetables and weight management, the best advice is to eat more. For this reason, there are no limits on portions of the vegetables in Energy Density Category 1—eat all that you like, raw or cooked with little to no fat. Included are all but the starchy vegetables such as corn, peas, potatoes, squash, and yams, as well as oil-containing vegetables such as olives and avocados. Such Category 2 vegetables should be part of your plan, but pay attention to portions. You shouldn't think of giving up starchy vegetables—they are rich in nutrients and can boost your fiber intake.

Remember that unlimited portions for vegetables are acceptable only if you do not add fat. Vegetables can be fat sponges when you cook them. To keep vegetables low in fat, cook mushrooms, onions, garlic, celery, and other veggies in bouillon, low-fat chicken broth, or a small amount of wine, instead of butter, margarine, or oil. Brown vegetables and meats separately, so the vegetables do not absorb fat from the meat. Instead of relying on added fat for flavor, try herbs and seasonings.

Go for variety when it comes to vegetables. Different types of produce contain different nutrients. It seems as if new health benefits from vegetables and fruits are being discovered every day. To ensure you are maximizing the nutritional benefits, choose a variety of colors of produce, especially those that are deeply colored. They contain a wide range of vitamins, minerals, fiber, antioxidants, and phytonutrients your body needs to maintain optimal health, protect against the effects of aging, and reduce the risk of cancer and heart disease. To learn more about the benefits of eating vegetables (and fruits), visit the website for the Produce for Better Health Foundation at www.5aday.org.

When you are in a hurry, don't skimp on vegetables—there are so many convenient ways to sneak them in to your day. We have developed some delicious vegetable side dishes and vegetarian entrées that will help you feel full and satisfied.

Here are some ways to sneak extra vegetables into your day.

- Learn to love your microwave. Many vegetables will cook in just a few minutes. For example, fresh asparagus with a little water and a squeeze of lemon, takes only 2 or 3 minutes on high power in a covered dish.
- Snack on baby carrots, celery sticks, or grape tomatoes at work.
- Add tomatoes, radishes, celery, and bell peppers to tuna or chicken salad.
- At your next barbecue, put vegetables such as zucchini, yellow squash, onions, cherry tomatoes, or mushrooms on skewers. A light coating of oil will add flavor and keep them from burning.
- Top broiled chicken or fish with Tex-Mex Salsa (page 78).
- Buy ready-to-eat, cleaned salad greens, or head to a salad bar and take prepared vegetables home for dinner.
- Stock your kitchen with vegetables that keep well, such as onions, scallions, garlic, potatoes, squash, and carrots. Pick up more perishable items like lettuce more frequently.
- Practice preventative eating: Have cut-up veggies handy on a plate with low-fat dressing, salsa, or hummus, and munch on them while you're making dinner, instead of reaching for a piece of cheese or chips. Both adults and kids are more likely to eat vegetables if they are already sliced.
- Add fresh, canned, or frozen vegetables to dishes you already like, such as pasta and pizza; add tomatoes, onions, cucumber, bell pepper, grated carrots, and dark-green lettuces, like romaine, to sandwiches.
- Add mushrooms to turn an ordinary dish into a treat. A cup of raw mushrooms adds only 20 calories.

Minted Broccoli

The mint and lemon juice complement the taste of broccoli, so it can be enjoyed without added fat. The energy density is so low you can eat as much as you like.

1 pound broccoli

¾ teaspoon salt

2 tablespoons lemon juice

Freshly ground black pepper

1 tablespoon chopped fresh mint

1. Remove the tough ends of the broccoli stems, peel the stems, and cut the broccoli into ½-inch-thick spears.

2. Bring 1 inch of water to a boil in a large saucepan. Add ½ teaspoon salt and the broccoli and simmer, covered, for 5 minutes. Drain the broccoli and return it to the pan.

3. Place the pan over very low heat. Sprinkle with the lemon juice, ¼ teaspoon of salt, a few grindings of black pepper, and the mint. Toss gently to combine.

YIELD: 4 servings of ¾ cup each

COOK'S NOTE: Try using your favorite fresh herb or combination of herbs in place of the mint.

Nutritional Information Per Serving

Calories 35 | Energy Density 0.28 | Carbohydrate 7 g. | Fat 1 g. | Protein 3 g. | Fiber 1 g.

For a 20-calorie side dish

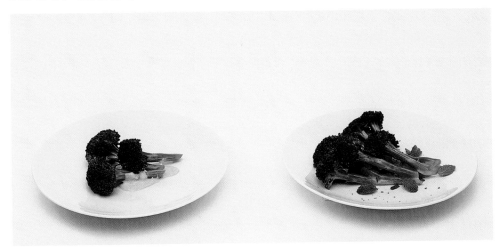

TRADITIONAL	How we lowered the ED	VOLUMETRICS
Broccoli with cheese sauce	▸ Omitted cheese sauce ▸ Used fresh herbs for flavor	Minted Broccoli

Garlic-Roasted Vegetables

Roasting slightly caramelizes the vegetables and brings out their full flavor in this side dish.

1 cup cauliflowerettes
1 cup broccoli florets
2 cups 1-inch-thick slices of zucchini
1½ cups 1-inch-long carrot sticks
1½ cups thickly sliced onions
1½ cups unpeeled boiling potatoes, cut into
   1-inch cubes

1 teaspoon chopped garlic
1 teaspoon dried thyme
½ teaspoon salt
¼ teaspoon freshly ground black pepper
¼ cup chopped, fresh flat-leaf parsley

1. Preheat the oven to 400 degrees.

2. Lightly coat a 9-by-13-inch baking dish with cooking spray.

3. Place all the ingredients, except the parsley, in the baking dish and toss well. Arrange in an even layer and lightly coat with cooking spray. Bake for 40 to 45 minutes, or until potatoes are tender.

4. Serve sprinkled with the parsley.

YIELD: 4 servings of 1¾ cups each

COOK'S NOTE: Other vegetables, such as bell peppers, yellow squash, or eggplant can be substituted for the cauliflower and broccoli. Experiment with your favorites.

Nutritional Information Per Serving

Calories 90 | Energy Density 0.40 | Carbohydrate 19 g. | Fat 1 g. | Protein 3 g. | Fiber 4 g.

For a 90-calorie side dish

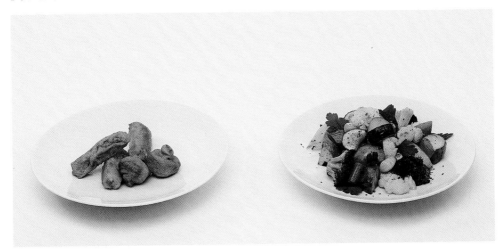

TRADITIONAL	How we lowered the ED	VOLUMETRICS
Breaded deep-fried vegetables	▸ Omitted the breading ▸ Oven-roasted instead of deep fried ▸ Used garlic for flavor	Garlic-Roasted Vegetables

Ratatouille

This quick-to-prepare version of the versatile classic French recipe makes a flavorful side dish. It can be served hot or at room temperature. Try it as a dip, a topping for pasta and baked potatoes, or a filling for omelets.

1 tablespoon extra-virgin olive oil
1 cup diced zucchini
1 cup unpeeled, diced eggplant
½ cup halved and sliced onions
1 teaspoon chopped garlic
1½ cups canned diced tomatoes, with liquid

½ cup vegetable broth
2 tablespoons tomato paste
¼ teaspoon salt
¼ teaspoon freshly ground black pepper
2 tablespoons chopped fresh basil

1. Heat the oil in a 12" nonstick skillet over medium-high heat. Add the zucchini, eggplant, onions, and garlic and cook, stirring occasionally, 5 minutes.

2. Add the rest of the ingredients, except the basil, and bring to a simmer, stirring. Cook 10 minutes, stirring occasionally. Stir in the basil and serve.

YIELD: 4 servings of ¾ cup each

Nutritional Information Per Serving

Calories 75 | Energy Density 0.50 | Carbohydrate 9 g. | Fat 4 g. | Protein 2 g. | Fiber 2 g.

Roasted Asparagus

Roasting gives the asparagus in this side dish a deep, mellow flavor. Pictured on page 4.

1½ pounds thick asparagus spears
Salt

Freshly ground black pepper
2 tablespoons grated Parmesan cheese

1. Preheat the oven to 400 degrees.

2. Lightly coat a baking sheet with cooking spray.

3. Break off the tough root ends of the asparagus. Peel off the tough skin with a paring knife. Place on the baking sheet in single layer. Lightly spray the asparagus with cooking spray. Season lightly with the salt and pepper. Sprinkle evenly with the Parmesan and roast for 15 minutes, or until tender when pierced with the tip of a knife.

YIELD: 4 servings of ¾ cup each

COOK'S NOTE: Thicker asparagus spears work best in this recipe. If using thin spears, shorten the baking time to about 10 minutes. Parmesan can be omitted, if desired.

Nutritional Information Per Serving

Calories 50 | Energy Density 0.40 | Carbohydrate 8 g. | Fat 1 g. | Protein 5 g. | Fiber 4 g.

Stir-Fried Green Beans

Stir-frying is a way to quickly prepare dishes with fresh, crisp textures and flavors using only a little fat. Notice the low energy density of these beans!

1½ teaspoons sesame oil
1½ pounds green beans, trimmed and cut
  into 1-inch pieces

1½ teaspoons reduced-sodium soy sauce
1 teaspoon sugar

1. Heat the oil over medium-high heat in a large nonstick skillet or wok. Add the green beans and stir-fry 3 minutes. Add the soy sauce and stir-fry 1 minute. Add the sugar and stir-fry 30 seconds.

YIELD: 4 servings of 1¼ cups each

COOK'S NOTE: Thin asparagus can be substituted for the green beans. Sliced bamboo shoots provide an attractive garnish.

Nutritional Information Per Serving

Calories 65 | Energy Density 0.40 | Carbohydrate 12 g. | Fat 2 g. | Protein 3 g. | Fiber 5 g.

For a 65-calorie side dish

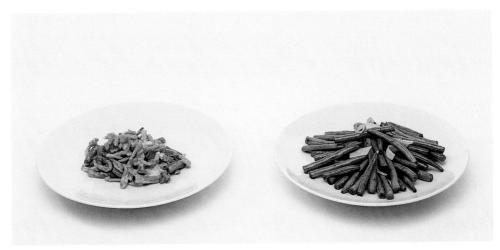

TRADITIONAL	How we lowered the ED	VOLUMETRICS
Green-bean casserole	▸ Omitted cream soup ▸ Omitted fried onions ▸ Used a small amount of sesame oil to increase flavor	Stir-Fried Green Beans

Crisp Stir-Fried Vegetables

Stir-frying this hearty vegetarian entrée retains the full flavor of the vegetables with little fat.

⅓ cup reduced-sodium soy sauce

2 tablespoons rice-wine vinegar

2 teaspoons sesame oil

4 teaspoons cornstarch

1 tablespoon vegetable oil

1 tablespoon minced fresh ginger

1 tablespoon minced garlic

2 cups broccoli florets

2 cups snow peas

1 cup seeded, thinly sliced, red or green bell peppers

2 cups sliced mushrooms, about ½ pound

2 cups fresh bean sprouts

1 cup peeled, grated carrots

1 cup canned water chestnuts, rinsed and drained

1 cup canned bamboo shoots, rinsed and drained

1 cup canned baby corn, rinsed and drained

3 cups cooked brown basmati rice

1. In a small bowl, combine the soy sauce, vinegar, sesame oil, and cornstarch and set aside.

2. Heat the vegetable oil in a large nonstick skillet or wok over medium-high heat. When the oil is hot, add the ginger and garlic and stir-fry 1 minute. Add the broccoli and snow peas to the skillet and stir-fry 3 minutes. Add the bell peppers, mushrooms, sprouts, carrots, water chestnuts, bamboo shoots, and baby corn, and stir-fry 3 minutes.

3. Stir the sauce, add it to the skillet, and stir-fry 1 minute, or until the sauce thickens. Divide the rice and stir-fry among 4 plates.

YIELD: 4 servings of ¾ cup rice and 2 cups stir-fry each

Nutritional Information Per Serving

Calories 385 | Energy Density 0.80 | Carbohydrate 66 g. | Fat 9 g. | Protein 14 g. | Fiber 12 g.

Tofu Pad Thai

Tofu or bean curd stands in for meat in many vegetarian dishes. It absorbs flavors of the sauce in which it is cooking.

6 ounces Asian rice noodles

1 cup vegetable broth

2 tablespoons bottled fish sauce

1 tablespoon rice-wine vinegar

1 tablespoon lime juice

3 tablespoons tomato paste

1 tablespoon sugar

½ tablespoon seeded, minced jalapeño

1 tablespoon peanut oil

1 teaspoon garlic

1 egg

8 ounces extra-firm tofu, diced into ¼-inch cubes

1 cup chopped onions

2½ cups fresh bean sprouts

½ cup chopped fresh cilantro

¼ cup chopped, dry-roasted peanuts

4 cups shredded romaine lettuce

1. Prepare the noodles as directed on the package.

2. In a small bowl, combine the broth, sauce, vinegar, lime juice, tomato paste, sugar, and jalapeño and set aside.

3. In a large nonstick skillet or a wok, heat the oil over medium heat and sauté the garlic. Add the egg and scramble it into small pieces. Increase the heat to high, add the tofu, and sauté 2 minutes, stirring gently. Add the sauce mixture and cook 1 minute, or until it comes to a boil.

4. Reduce the heat to medium, and add the rice noodles, onions, sprouts, cilantro, and peanuts to the skillet. Heat thoroughly while tossing until the noodles are coated.

5. Divide the romaine among 4 plates and serve the Pad Thai over it.

YIELD: 4 servings of 2 cups each

COOK'S NOTE: For a vegetarian dish, substitute soy sauce for the fish sauce.

Nutritional Information Per Serving

Calories 375 | Energy Density 0.90 | Carbohydrate 52 g. | Fat 14 g. | Protein 15 g. | Fiber 4 g.

New Potatoes with Peas

Mint enlivens the flavor of these potatoes, creating a very pleasant-tasting side dish.

¾ *pound scrubbed, unpeeled small new potatoes*

8 *scallions, trimmed, white part left whole, green part chopped*

1½ *cups frozen peas, unthawed*

1 *teaspoon unsalted butter*

1 *tablespoon chopped fresh mint*

Freshly ground black pepper

1. Place the potatoes and white parts of the scallions in a medium saucepan and cover with water. Bring to a simmer and cook 15 to 20 minutes, or until the potatoes are tender when pierced with the tip of a knife.

2. Add the peas and cook 4 minutes over medium heat. Drain the potatoes, scallions, and peas and return to the pan. Add the butter, mint, and a few grindings of pepper. Heat the mixture, over very low heat, 1 minute. Toss gently with the chopped green scallions.

YIELD: 4 servings of 1 cup each

COOK'S NOTE: If new potatoes are not available, substitute unpeeled white boiling potatoes cut into 1-inch cubes.

Nutritional Information Per Serving

Calories 135 | Energy Density 0.80 | Carbohydrate 26 g. | Fat 1 g. | Protein 5 g. | Fiber 5 g.

Oven-Roasted Potatoes

This side dish is a delicious, low-fat alternative to deep-fried potatoes.

1¼ pounds unpeeled, medium red-skinned
    potatoes, each cut into 8 wedges
½ teaspoon dried thyme

Salt
Freshly ground black pepper
¼ cup chopped fresh parsley

1. Preheat the oven to 400 degrees.

2. Lightly coat a baking dish with cooking spray and add the potatoes, skin side down. Spray the potatoes lightly with cooking spray. Sprinkle the potatoes with thyme and season lightly with the salt and pepper. Roast the potatoes 40 minutes.

3. Serve the potatoes sprinkled with the parsley.

YIELD: 4 servings of ⅔ cup each

COOK'S NOTE: Any boiling potato can be substituted for the red skins. For a Cajun flavor, add 2 teaspoons chili powder and ¼ teaspoon cayenne.

Nutritional Information Per Serving

Calories 110 | Energy Density 1.6 | Carbohydrate 24 g. | Fat 0 g. | Protein 3 g. | Fiber 2 g.

Smashed Potatoes

This lowered-fat version of mashed potatoes will provide just as much comfort as the usual dish, with fewer calories. Pictured on page 4.

*1½ pounds unpeeled, red-skinned potatoes
  cut into 1-inch cubes*
¼ cup nonfat milk

2 teaspoons unsalted butter
¼ teaspoon salt
¼ teaspoon freshly ground black pepper

1. Place the potatoes in a large saucepan, cover with water, and simmer 20 minutes, or until the potatoes are tender when pierced with the tip of a knife. Drain the potatoes, reserving ¼ cup cooking water. Return the potatoes to the saucepan and place over low heat.

2. Add the milk, butter, salt, and pepper. Mash with a potato masher until smooth. If the potatoes seem dry, stir in some of the reserved water.

YIELD: 4 servings of 1 cup each

COOK'S NOTE: For garlic potatoes, add 4 peeled cloves of garlic to the potatoes and water before simmering.

Nutritional Information Per Serving

Calories 155 | Energy Density 0.90 | Carbohydrate 32 g. | Fat 1 g. | Protein 3 g. | Fiber 2 g.

Herbed Barley Stuffed Squash

Acorn squash has a delicious nutty flavor and is packed with nutrients. The barley makes this a filling side dish.

2 acorn squash, halved and seeded
1½ cups cooked barley
½ cup chopped scallions
½ cup finely chopped celery
2 tablespoons toasted pine nuts (page 84)

2 tablespoons chopped fresh marjoram
2 teaspoons extra-virgin olive oil
½ teaspoon salt
¼ teaspoon freshly ground black pepper
1 teaspoon paprika

1. Preheat the oven to 350 degrees. Coat a baking sheet with cooking spray.

2. Place the squash, cut sides up, on the baking sheet and bake 25 minutes.

3. Combine the barley, scallions, celery, pine nuts, marjoram, oil, salt, and pepper in a medium bowl. Divide this mixture among the cavities of each squash half. Sprinkle with the paprika and bake 20 to 25 minutes, or until the squash is tender.

YIELD: 4 servings

Nutritional Information Per Serving

Calories 210 | Energy Density 0.60 | Carbohydrate 41 g. | Fat 5 g. | Protein 4 g. | Fiber 6 g.

Bulgur and Vegetable Stuffed Peppers

Bulgur provides the extra fiber associated with whole grains, and gives this dish a hearty texture. Enjoy this as a side dish, or double the portion to make a main dish.

1 cup vegetable broth
⅔ cup bulgur
4 red, yellow, or orange bell peppers, about
   2 pounds
½ cup finely chopped celery
¼ cup chopped scallions
½ cup diced mushrooms, about 2 ounces

½ cup peeled, shredded carrots
¼ cup grated Parmesan cheese
½ teaspoon dried thyme
½ teaspoon dried oregano
½ teaspoon salt
Pinch cayenne

For a 150-calorie side dish

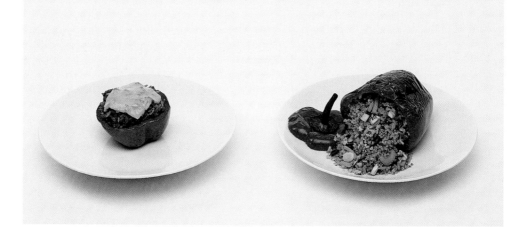

TRADITIONAL	How we lowered the ED	VOLUMETRICS
Sausage-stuffed peppers	▸ Decreased amount of oil ▸ Omitted sausage ▸ Added bulgur and vegetables	Bulgur and Vegetable Stuffed Peppers

1. Bring the broth and bulgur to a boil in a 2-quart saucepan, stirring constantly. Reduce the heat and simmer, covered, 10 minutes. Fluff with a fork and put in a large bowl.

2. Preheat the oven to 375 degrees.

3. Lightly coat an 8-by-8-inch baking dish with cooking spray.

4. Cut the tops off the bell peppers and remove the core and seeds. Cut a very thin slice off the bottom of the bell peppers so they will stand upright.

5. Cook the peppers, in a large pot of boiling water, 3 minutes. Remove the peppers and drain, inverted, on paper towels.

6. Combine the remaining ingredients with the bulgur. Divide the mixture among the peppers. Place the peppers upright in the baking dish and bake 15 to 20 minutes.

YIELD: 4 servings

COOK'S NOTE: Bulgur is available in the natural-food section of some supermarkets and in specialty grocery stores.

Nutritional Information Per Serving

Calories 150 | Energy Density 0.50 | Carbohydrate 27 g. | Fat 3 g. | Protein 8 g. | Fiber 8 g.

Chickpea Curry

Chickpeas, or garbanzo beans, add lots of nutrients and fiber to this spicy vegetarian main dish.

1 tablespoon extra-virgin olive oil

1 cup chopped onions

1½ teaspoons chopped garlic

1½ teaspoons chopped fresh ginger

1½ teaspoons curry powder

½ teaspoon ground turmeric

⅛ teaspoon crushed red-pepper flakes

½ teaspoon salt

4 cups cored, chopped tomatoes

1½ teaspoons sugar

3 cups canned chickpeas, rinsed and drained

1½ cups baby spinach

1½ cups small cauliflowerettes

½ teaspoon garam masala

3 cups cooked brown basmati rice

1. Heat the oil in a 4- to 5-quart pan over medium heat. Add the onions and sauté 5 minutes. Stir in the garlic, ginger, curry powder, turmeric, red-pepper flakes, and salt. Cook 2 minutes, stirring.

2. Stir in the tomatoes and sugar and cook on medium-low heat 10 minutes, stirring occasionally.

3. Stir in the chickpeas, spinach, cauliflower, and garam masala. Simmer, covered, 10 minutes, stirring occasionally.

4. Divide the rice and curry among 6 bowls.

YIELD: 6 servings of 1 cup of curry and ½ cup rice each

COOK'S NOTE: Garam masala is an Indian spice blend that can be found in the spice section of large supermarkets and in specialty grocery stores.

Nutritional Information Per Serving

Calories 325 | Energy Density 0.70 | Carbohydrate 61 g. | Fat 5 g. | Protein 11 g. | Fiber 10 g.

Eggplant "Lasagna"

In this vegetarian main dish, replacing the lasagna noodles with eggplant slices lowers the energy density while giving a new twist to lasagna.

¾ cup breadcrumbs (see Cook's Note)

2 tablespoons grated Parmesan cheese

2 teaspoons dried oregano

2 eggs

2 medium eggplant, peeled and cut cross-wise into ¼-inch slices, about 2 pounds

1¾ cups Tomato and Fresh Basil Sauce (page 233)

1 cup shredded 2 percent fat mozzarella cheese

1. Preheat the oven to 400 degrees.

2. Combine the breadcrumbs, Parmesan, and oregano in a shallow bowl.

3. Beat the eggs with 2 tablespoons water in a shallow bowl.

4. Dredge the eggplant slices in the egg mixture, then lightly coat them with the breadcrumb mixture. Place the eggplant slices on a baking sheet and bake, turning once, 20 to 30 minutes, or until browned. Allow to cool slightly.

5. Spread ¾ cup of the tomato sauce on the bottom of a 9-by-9-inch casserole dish. Arrange half of the eggplant slices on top of the sauce. Cover with ½ cup tomato sauce and ½ cup mozzarella.

6. Repeat with the remaining eggplant, tomato sauce, and mozzarella.

7. Cover and bake 30 minutes. Take the cover off and bake an additional 15 minutes.

YIELD: 4 servings, each 4½" by 4½"

COOK'S NOTE: Make breadcrumbs by pulverizing torn pieces of bread in a food processor or blender.

Nutritional Information Per Serving

Calories 355 | Energy Density 1.1 | Carbohydrate 43 g. | Fat 12 g. | Protein 19 g. | Fiber 7 g.

Classic Vegetarian Vegetable Stew

Roasted vegetables and brown rice make this stew a filling entrée.

1 cup thickly sliced onions
2 cups peeled 1-inch turnip pieces
1 cup 1-inch celery pieces
1 cup peeled 1-inch carrot pieces
1 cup 1-inch cube peeled boiling potatoes
2 cups ¼-inch-thick slices leeks
1 cup peeled 1-inch parsnips pieces
1 tablespoon extra-virgin olive oil
2 sprigs each fresh thyme and fresh
   parsley or other fresh herbs

2 cups vegetable broth
1¾ cups canned diced tomatoes, undrained
1 bay leaf
2 teaspoons chopped garlic
2 cups shredded Swiss chard, tough stems
   removed
Salt
Freshly ground black pepper
2 cups cooked brown rice

1. Preheat the oven to 475 degrees.

2. Combine the onions, turnips, celery, carrots, potatoes, leek, parsnips, and oil in a roasting pan and toss to coat the vegetables with the oil. Roast 30 minutes, stirring twice.

3. Tie the herb sprigs together with kitchen string.

4. Transfer the vegetables to a large pot and heat over medium-high heat. Stir in the broth, tomatoes, bay leaf, garlic, herb bundle, and 1½ cups water and cook 15 minutes, stirring occasionally.

5. Stir in the chard, season lightly with salt and pepper, and cook 2 minutes. Remove the bay leaf and herb bundle.

6. Serve the stew over the rice in 4 shallow bowls.

YIELD: 4 servings of ¾ cup stew and ½ cup rice each

COOK'S NOTE: Winter squash, such as acorn or butternut, can be substituted for the parsnips or turnips. Other leafy green vegetables such as spinach, collard greens, or kale can be used in place of the chard. For another version of vegetable stew, start with Garlic-Roasted Vegetables (page 160). After roasting, proceed as directed.

Nutritional Information Per Serving

Calories 270 | Energy Density 0.60 | Carbohydrate 50 g. | Fat 6 g. | Protein 8 g. | Fiber 8 g.

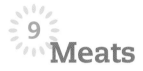

9 Meats

Chapters 9, 10, and 11 feature recipes for delicious entrées based on protein-rich meats, fish, and poultry. Unless you are a vegetarian, it is likely that you will plan at least one meal a day around such entrées. Some of you, having heard that protein speeds weight loss, may be eating more meat. That is okay as long as you choose lean or lower-fat meat—you already know that, because of its high energy density, fat packs in the calories. You also should know that numerous studies have found that eating large amounts of animal fat is related to heart disease.

What we do not yet know is whether protein helps with weight loss in the long term. Several studies have shown that people who ate a high-protein diet for six months lost more weight than people who followed a diet lower in protein. However, over the next six months, the lost weight started to return and the difference between the groups disappeared. Maintaining lost weight is always the most difficult part of weight management and can only be successful when healthy eating and physical activity become a part of your life.

Protein may help with weight loss by increasing satiety and keeping hunger under control. Several studies have shown that increasing protein intake led to increased fullness. Part of this satiety effect could be psychological, since meals are often thought to be more complete or substantial if they contain meat or other high-protein entrées.

You can use the satiating power of protein to manage your weight by eating adequate amounts of lean protein. Whether we are meat eaters or vegetarians, most of us are eating plenty of protein. The amount of protein you need each day is based on your body weight. The usual recommendation is 0.4 grams per pound of body weight. If you are very active, you can go up to 0.8 grams per pound.

Let's consider how you can make smart meat choices. Generally, portions are too large. Eat an 8-ounce sirloin steak and you will get around 600 calories and from 30 to 40 grams of fat. The recommended portion of red meat is 2 to 3 ounces, around the size of a deck of cards. Such portions of lean red meat can fit into a healthy *Volumetrics* diet. But how do you know which cuts are lean and which are higher in saturated fat? Here are some tips.

- Hamburger meat is the biggest contributor of saturated fat to the American diet. Even if it is labeled "lean" you should cook hamburger so the fat drips off or can be removed. But the fat loss during cooking does not turn a fatty burger into a lean burger, so choose 97, 95, or 90 percent lean beef.
- Trim fat from meat and choose cuts with the least marbling.
- Some of the leanest cuts of beef are round and loin.
- The leanest pork is from tenderloin, top loin roast, or chops, or Canadian bacon.
- Lean lamb includes roasts and chops.
- Look at the grade of beef: prime has the most fat, choice is next, and select has the least.
- Choose low-fat deli meats, sausages, and hot dogs.

The recipes that I have included give you meat dishes that will leave you full and satisfied without a lot of fat or calories.

Stir-Fried Beef with Snow Peas and Tomatoes

This mildly spicy main dish is a good choice when you need to get dinner on the table quickly.

1 pound well-trimmed flank steak

1 tablespoon cornstarch

1 tablespoon reduced-sodium soy sauce

1 tablespoon minced fresh ginger

1 teaspoon sugar

1 tablespoon vegetable oil

3 scallions, cut in 1-inch lengths

1½ teaspoons minced garlic

6 ounces snow peas

2 cups cored, chopped tomatoes

¼ teaspoon hot-pepper sauce

Freshly ground black pepper

1. Cut the beef in half lengthwise and slice it thinly across the grain.

2. Combine the cornstarch, soy sauce, ginger, and ½ teaspoon sugar in a large bowl. Stir until smooth. Add the beef and toss well.

3. Heat 1½ teaspoons oil in a large nonstick skillet or wok over moderately high heat. Add half of the beef, stir-fry 2 minutes. Transfer the beef to a plate with a slotted spoon. Repeat with the remaining 1½ teaspoons oil and remaining beef. Set the beef aside.

4. Add the scallions, garlic, snow peas, tomatoes, the remaining ½ teaspoon sugar, and hot-pepper sauce and stir-fry 3 minutes. Return the beef and any liquid on the plate to the skillet and stir-fry 1 minute. Add a few grindings of black pepper and stir again.

YIELD: 4 servings of 1½ cups each

COOK'S NOTE: Green beans cut into 1-inch pieces or sugar snap peas can be substituted for the snow peas. This is good served with boiled brown rice.

Nutritional Information Per Serving

Calories 255 | Energy Density 1.2 | Carbohydrate 11 g. | Fat 12 g. | Protein 26 g. | Fiber 2 g.

Old World Goulash

This volumetric version of the traditional Hungarian beef stew provides satisfying portions with lots of vegetables.

1 tablespoon extra-virgin olive oil

1 pound well-trimmed, boneless beef
  round roast, cut into 1-inch pieces

½ teaspoon salt

¼ teaspoon freshly ground black pepper

1 cup chopped onions

1 teaspoon chopped garlic

2 cups sliced mushrooms, about ⅓ pound

1 cup nonfat, reduced-sodium beef broth

2 cups peeled, diced boiling potatoes, about
  1 pound

2 cups peeled, thinly sliced carrots

1 cup sliced celery

12 ounces trimmed green beans,
  cut into 1-inch lengths

2 tablespoons paprika

½ teaspoon dried thyme

1 tablespoon tomato paste

2 tablespoons cornstarch

2 tablespoons dry red wine

1. Lightly coat a 4- to 5-quart heavy pot or Dutch oven with cooking spray. Add the oil and heat over medium-high heat. Add the beef, salt, and pepper. Cook, stirring occasionally, until the beef browns, 6 to 8 minutes.

2. Add the onions, garlic, and mushrooms and cook 5 minutes.

3. Add the broth, and enough water to barely cover the ingredients in the pot. Bring to a simmer, stirring occasionally. Cover the pot and cook 45 minutes, stirring occasionally.

4. Add the potatoes, carrots, celery, beans, paprika, thyme, and tomato paste and stir well. Add more water, if necessary, to barely cover. Simmer, uncovered, 45 minutes, stirring occasionally. Add additional water, if necessary, to prevent the stew from drying out.

5. Whisk the cornstarch and wine in a small bowl until smooth. Stir the mixture into the goulash and cook over medium-high heat, stirring occasionally, until slightly thickened and bubbly, about 3 minutes. Taste the sauce and season with salt and pepper, if necessary.

YIELD: 4 servings of 2½ cups each

COOK'S NOTE: The paprika provides the distinctive flavor and color of this dish so be sure it is fresh. The goulash is delicious by itself, but it is often served with noodles. Try whole-wheat, broad egg noodles, or short pasta such as whole-wheat fusilli or penne.

Nutritional Information Per Serving

Calories 335 | Energy Density 0.60 | Carbohydrate 32 g. | Fat 11 g. | Protein 30 g. | Fiber 10 g.

For a 335-calorie entrée

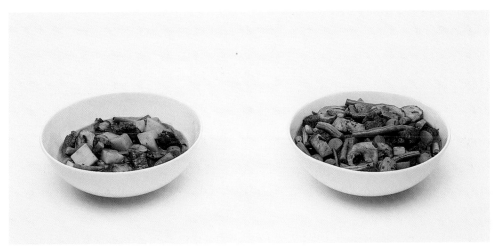

TRADITIONAL	How we lowered the ED	VOLUMETRICS
Traditional beef goulash	▸ Used less oil to sauté ▸ Omitted sour cream ▸ Used lean beef and twice as many vegetables	Old World Goulash

Shepherd's Pie

A pie that's not a real pie, this is a traditional pub favorite in England and Ireland. My fragrant main dish version includes the usual meat and mashed potatoes, but is loaded with volumetric vegetables.

1½ teaspoons extra-virgin olive oil
½ cup diced celery
½ cup diced onions
1½ teaspoons minced garlic
2 tablespoons flour
1 pound 95 percent lean ground beef
1½ cups nonfat, reduced-sodium beef broth
1½ cups canned diced tomatoes, with liquid
¼ cup tomato paste

½ teaspoon dried thyme
½ teaspoon freshly ground black pepper
2 teaspoons minced garlic
¼ teaspoon paprika
¼ teaspoon salt
1 cup sliced mushrooms, about 4 ounces
1 cup peeled, sliced carrots
½ cup frozen baby peas, thawed
½ cup frozen corn, thawed
Smashed Potatoes (page 170)
¼ cup shredded low-fat Cheddar cheese

1. Preheat the oven to 375 degrees.

2. Heat the oil in a large skillet over medium heat. Add the celery, onions, and garlic and sauté until the vegetables are slightly tender, about 5 minutes. Add the flour and continue cooking, stirring constantly, 2 minutes. Remove the vegetables from the pan.

3. In the same pan, cook the beef over medium heat until no longer pink. Drain any visible fat.

4. Add the celery mixture to the beef. Add the broth, tomatoes, tomato paste, thyme, pepper, garlic, paprika, and salt and stir well. Cook the mixture 5 minutes, or until slightly thickened. Reduce the heat to medium-low and stir in the mushrooms, carrots, peas, and corn. Simmer the mixture 10 to 15 minutes.

5. Pour the beef mixture into a 3- to 4-quart casserole dish. Spread the Smashed Potatoes evenly over the top of the beef mixture and sprinkle with Cheddar.

6. Bake the casserole, uncovered, 30 to 40 minutes, or until bubbly.

7. Remove the casserole from the oven and preheat the broiler.

8. Broil the casserole 1 minute, or until the cheese is lightly browned.

YIELD: 6 servings of 1½ cups each

Nutritional Information Per Serving

Calories 315 | Energy Density 0.90 | Carbohydrate 36 g. | Fat 8 g. | Protein 25 g. | Fiber 3 g.

Nouveau Lamb Stew

I updated this satisfying main dish by decreasing the calories and fat and adding Mediterranean-inspired flavors.

1 teaspoon extra-virgin olive oil

1 pound boneless lamb shoulder, excess fat removed, cut in 1-inch pieces

1 cup chopped onions

½ teaspoon salt

Pinch freshly ground black pepper

1 cup nonfat, reduced-sodium beef broth

1½ cups peeled, diced boiling potatoes

2 cups peeled, chopped turnips

1 cup peeled, thickly sliced carrots

1 cup sliced celery

½ teaspoon dried thyme

½ teaspoon chopped garlic

2 tablespoons cornstarch

2 tablespoons dry red wine

1 cup frozen peas, thawed

For a 245-calorie entrée

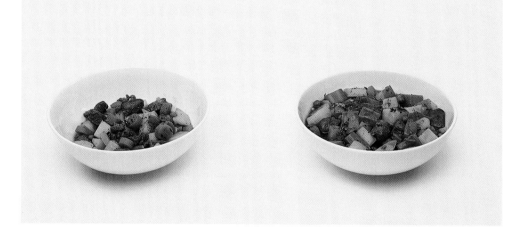

TRADITIONAL	How we lowered the ED	VOLUMETRICS
Lamb stew	▸ Decreased oil ▸ Used less meat and trimmed all visible fat ▸ Doubled the amount of veggies	Nouveau Lamb Stew

1. Lightly coat a 4- to 5-quart heavy pot or Dutch oven with cooking spray. Add the oil and heat over medium-high heat.

2. Add the lamb, and cook, stirring occasionally, until the lamb is lightly browned. Stir in the onions, salt, and pepper and cook 5 minutes. Add the broth and enough water to cover the meat. Bring to a simmer, stirring occasionally. Cover the pot and cook 1 hour, stirring occasionally.

3. Add the potatoes, turnips, carrots, celery, thyme, and garlic. Add more water, if necessary, to barely cover all the ingredients. Bring back to a simmer, stirring, and cook, uncovered, 30 minutes.

4. Whisk the cornstarch and wine in a small bowl until smooth. Stir the cornstarch mixture and peas into the stew. Raise the heat to medium-high and cook, stirring, until slightly thickened and bubbly, about 3 minutes. Taste for seasoning and, if desired, add more salt and pepper.

YIELD: 4 servings of 2½ cups each

COOK'S NOTE: This stew is even better reheated. Cool, cover, and place in the refrigerator overnight. Remove any fat that settles on the surface. Return to the stove and cook, stirring occasionally, over medium heat, until bubbly.

Nutritional Information Per Serving

Calories 245 | Energy Density 0.40 | Carbohydrate 28 g. | Fat 6 g. | Protein 20 g. | Fiber 6 g.

Pork Chops with Orange-Soy Sauce

The orange juice and soy sauce reduction makes a great tasting sauce. This main dish can be prepared quickly enough to make any night a special occasion.

1 cup orange juice

1 tablespoon reduced-sodium soy sauce

2 teaspoons minced garlic

½ teaspoon dried thyme

4 pork chops, 4- to 6-ounces each, trimmed of fat

Salt

Freshly ground black pepper

1 tablespoon vegetable oil

For a 195-calorie entrée

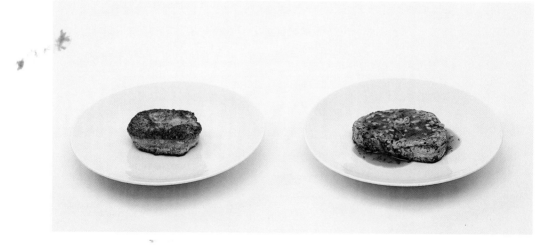

TRADITIONAL	How we lowered the ED	VOLUMETRICS
Breaded and fried pork chops	▸ Omitted breading ▸ Instead of pan frying, browned chop with a small amount of oil and finished it in the oven ▸ Added sauce for flavor	Pork Chops with Orange-Soy Sauce

1. Preheat the oven to 400 degrees.

2. Combine the juice, soy sauce, garlic, and thyme in a small bowl and set aside.

3. Lightly season the pork chops with salt and pepper.

4. Heat the oil in a large skillet over high heat. Add the pork chops and brown 3 minutes per side. Transfer the chops to a baking dish and bake 10 to 15 minutes, or until no longer pink.

5. Remove any fat from the skillet. Add the orange-soy mixture to the skillet and cook, stirring, over high heat, 3 to 5 minutes, or until reduced by half. Return the chops and any juices to the skillet and heat through, turning once.

YIELD: 4 servings

Nutritional Information Per Serving

Calories 195 | Energy Density 1.6 | Carbohydrate 7 g. | Fat 9 g. | Protein 20 g. | Fiber 1 g.

Roasted Lamb Chops with Gremolata

The quick roasting produces a juicy meat entrée that is full of flavor. It is finished with a lively mixture of parsley, garlic, and lemon zest called gremolata.

4 well-trimmed, 1-inch thick, loin lamb
   chops, about 4 ounces each
1 garlic clove, halved
1 teaspoon extra-virgin olive oil
Salt

Freshly ground black pepper
¼ cup chopped, fresh flat-leaf parsley
1 teaspoon chopped garlic
1 teaspoon grated lemon zest

1. Preheat the oven to 450 degrees.

2. Rub both sides of the chops with the cut sides of the garlic cloves. Lightly brush the chops on both sides with oil. Lightly season the chops on both sides with salt and pepper.

3. Heat a large oven-safe nonstick skillet over high heat. Add the chops and cook 2 minutes. Turn the chops over and place the skillet in the oven. Roast 8 to 10 minutes for medium rare.

4. Prepare the gremolata by combining the parsley, chopped garlic, and lemon zest in a small bowl. Set aside.

5. Divide the chops among 4 warmed plates. Sprinkle 1 tablespoon gremolata on each.

YIELD: 4 servings

COOK'S NOTE: This method works equally well with tender, well-trimmed cuts of 1-inch-thick beefsteak. If you do not have an oven-safe skillet, wrap the skillet handle in aluminum foil before placing it in the oven.

Nutritional Information Per Serving

Calories 140 | Energy Density 1.3 | Carbohydrate 1 g. | Fat 6 g. | Protein 19 g. | Fiber 1 g.

10 Fish and Shellfish

The fat content and energy density of different types of fish and shellfish vary widely. In general, the lighter the color of the flesh, the lower the fat content. For example, white fish such as cod, flounder, fresh tuna, and orange roughy have about 1 to 2 grams of fat per 4 ounces. Pale-colored fish such as pink salmon, catfish, halibut, and swordfish have 3 to 6 grams of fat per 4 ounces, and dark fish such as mackerel, rainbow trout, herring, and red tuna range from 8 to 16 grams of fat per 4 ounces. Unlike the saturated fat found in red meat, the oil in fish provides important health benefits. These omega-3 fatty acids are also found in some shellfish, such as scallops. A recent statement from the American Heart Association confirms that omega-3 fatty acids reduce the risk of heart disease. For this reason, they recommend eating at least 2 servings of fish (particularly fatty fish) per week. Remember that a serving is 2 to 3 ounces, or the size of a deck of cards.

Fish is an excellent example of why not all of your food choices should be made on the basis of calorie content or energy density alone. Nutritional balance is important—we eat not only to maintain our weight, but also to obtain the balance of nutrients required for optimal health. We need some fat in our diets, particularly the healthy fats that are found in fish, nuts, avocados, and olives. So go ahead and choose a fatty fish for heart health, and balance it with lots of vegetables. You can keep the calories moderate by grilling the fish or mixing it into dishes that do not require much additional fat, such as Fiesta Fish Stew (page 202).

For most people, the natural fat in fish should be much less of a worry than how they are preparing their fish. Fish that is battered and fried, or fish mixed with high-fat dressing, such as mayonnaise, is where the calories really add up.

Several other concerns have kept people away from fish. One is that some fish, such as swordfish, tuna, and mackerel, are contaminated with mercury. Children and pregnant women should limit their intake of these fish. The American Heart Association recommends eating a variety of fish to reduce any potentially harmful effects.

For years, some people have avoided shellfish, such as shrimp, because of their high cholesterol levels. It turns out that shrimp and clams are not as high in cholesterol as previously thought and, like other fish, they are low in saturated fat. Saturated fat is the real culprit in elevating blood cholesterol. So go ahead and enjoy shrimp, clams, and other shellfish. But, remember that the way the shellfish is prepared, especially if it is battered and fried, can affect the energy density.

You should be eating your fish for the healthy fats, and as an excellent source of protein. One more reason to choose fish is that it has been shown calorie for calorie to enhance satiety more than chicken or beef. After meals with the same amount of protein, people felt fuller following fish than chicken or beef. The *Volumetrics* recipes in this chapter will show you how easy it is to prepare delicious fish entrées.

Poach-Roast Salmon with Yogurt and Dill Sauce

This is a simple and almost foolproof method of cooking salmon fillets so that they remain moist.

½ cup nonfat plain yogurt
½ teaspoon minced garlic
1 tablespoon minced onions
1 tablespoon drained capers, chopped if large
3 tablespoons lemon juice

1 tablespoon chopped fresh dill
1 pound salmon fillet, cut crosswise into 4 equal portions
¼ teaspoon salt
Pinch freshly ground black pepper
4 lemon wedges

1. Preheat the oven to 400 degrees.

2. In a small bowl, stir the yogurt, garlic, onions, capers, 1 tablespoon lemon juice, and ½ tablespoon dill until smooth. Set the Yogurt and Dill Sauce aside.

3. Lightly coat an 8- by 12-inch glass baking dish with cooking spray.

4. Place the salmon, skin-side down, in the dish. Sprinkle with 2 tablespoons lemon juice. Season with salt, pepper, and ½ tablespoon dill. Cover the dish tightly with foil and bake 15 to 25 minutes until fish is flaky and no longer translucent.

5. Divide the salmon among 4 dinner plates and garnish with 2 tablespoons of the sauce and a lemon wedge.

YIELD: 4 servings

Nutritional Information Per Serving

Calories 225 | Energy Density 1.6 | Carbohydrate 4 g. | Fat 13 g. | Protein 24 g. | Fiber 0 g.

Nutritional Information Per Serving of Yogurt and Dill Sauce

Calories 15 | Energy Density 0.52 | Carbohydrate 2 g. | Fat 1 g. | Protein 1 g. | Fiber 1 g.

Baked Tilapia with Sautéed Vegetables

Try this simple method of cooking fish fillets for a colorful and delicious main dish.

1 to 1½ pounds tilapia fillets
½ cup orange juice
2 teaspoons vegetable oil
¼ teaspoon salt
1 cup chopped green bell peppers

¾ cup halved and sliced onions
2 teaspoons minced garlic
1½ cups canned diced tomatoes, with liquid

For a 160-calorie entrée

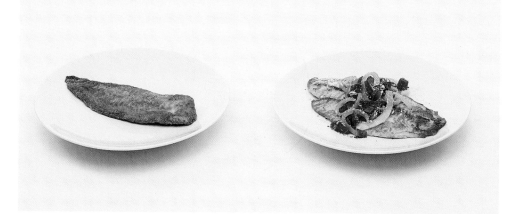

TRADITIONAL	How we lowered the ED	VOLUMETRICS
Breaded and fried fish	▸ Omitted the breading ▸ Baked the fish instead of frying ▸ Added vegetables	Baked Tilapia with Sautéed Vegetables

1. Preheat the oven to 350 degrees. Lightly coat a baking dish large enough to accommodate the fillets in one layer with cooking spray.

2. Rinse the fillets under cold water, pat dry, and place them in the baking dish in a single layer, skin side down.

3. Combine 2 tablespoons orange juice with 1 teaspoon oil and sprinkle over the fillets. Sprinkle with salt and bake 15 to 20 minutes, or until the fish is flaky and no longer translucent.

4. Lightly coat a large skillet with cooking spray, add remaining 1 teaspoon oil and heat over medium-high heat. Add the bell peppers and onions and cook, stirring occasionally, 5 minutes. Add the remaining orange juice, garlic, and tomatoes. Cook, stirring occasionally, 2 minutes, or until heated through.

5. Divide the fillets among 4 plates and spoon the sauce over them.

YIELD: 4 servings

COOK'S NOTE: Other fish choices are flounder, cod, red snapper, or sole. Lemon juice or dry white wine can be substituted for the orange juice. Try the Cherry Tomato Salsa (page 240) or the Mango Salsa (page 88) instead of the sautéed vegetables.

Nutritional Information Per Serving

Calories 160 | Energy Density 0.80 | Carbohydrate 10 g. | Fat 3 g. | Protein 22 g. | Fiber 2 g.

Sautéed Flounder with Lemon Sauce

The slight tartness of the lemon and caper sauce complements the flounder's delicate flavor.

⅓ cup all-purpose flour
½ teaspoon salt
Pinch freshly ground black pepper
1 tablespoon extra-virgin olive oil
1 pound flounder fillet
⅓ cup dry white wine
⅓ cup nonfat, reduced-sodium chicken broth

2 tablespoons lemon juice
1 tablespoon rinsed and drained capers
2 tablespoons chopped, fresh flat-leaf parsley
4 lemon wedges

1. Mix the flour, salt, and pepper in a shallow dish. Dredge the fillets in the flour mixture. Shake off excess.

2. Heat the oil in a large nonstick skillet over medium-high heat until hot. Place the fillets in the skillet and cook 4 minutes. Using a wide spatula, carefully turn the fillets over and cook another 4 minutes. Transfer the fillets to a plate, cover, and keep warm.

3. Add the wine, broth, and juice to the skillet. Stir, scraping up any crusty bits. Stir in the capers and bring to a simmer. Cook the sauce 1 minute, or until slightly reduced. Remove from the heat and stir in the parsley.

4. Divide the fillets, sauce, and lemon wedges among 4 dinner plates.

YIELD: 4 servings

COOK'S NOTE: Sole or tilapia fillets can be substituted for the flounder. Make sure that the skillet is hot before adding the fillets so that they brown properly. You can replace the wine with ⅓ cup chicken broth.

Nutritional Information Per Serving

Calories 180 | Energy Density 1.2 | Carbohydrate 7 g. | Fat 5 g. | Protein 23 g. | Fiber 1 g.

Fillet of Sole and Vegetable Parcels

Open these parcels at the table to allow the diner to enjoy the heady aroma of the contents.

2 medium zucchini, about ¾ pound
1 trimmed well-washed medium leek
½ pound trimmed thin asparagus
4 sole fillets, about 5 ounces each
4 tablespoons dry white wine

8 thin slices lemon
¼ cup chopped fresh dill
2 teaspoons chopped garlic
Salt
Freshly ground black pepper

1. Preheat the oven to 400 degrees.

2. Remove the ends of each zucchini. Using a broad vegetable peeler or mandolin, remove long, thin slices of the zucchini and set aside.

3. Cut the white part of the leek into julienne strips and the asparagus into 2-inch long pieces and set aside. Cut out 4 13-by-13-inch pieces of parchment paper.

4. Place 1 fillet on each of the parchment pieces. Sprinkle with the wine and top each with 2 lemon slices. Divide the zucchini, leeks, and asparagus over the fillets and sprinkle with the dill and garlic. Season lightly with salt and pepper.

5. Bring up the top and bottom sides of each piece of parchment paper and fold the edges over to form a tight seam. Twist the ends and tuck under the parcel.

6. Place the parcels on a baking sheet and bake 20 minutes. Serve the parcels unopened.

YIELD: 4 servings

COOK'S NOTE: Flounder or tilapia fillet can be substituted for the sole. Vegetable broth can be used in place of wine.

Nutritional Information Per Serving

Calories 230 | Energy Density 0.70 | Carbohydrate 9 g. | Fat 8 g. | Protein 30 g. | Fiber 3 g.

Jenny's Caribbean Tuna and Fruit Kebobs

Jenny, a Postdoctoral Fellow in my lab, created this main dish recipe after returning from a trip to Jamaica.

½ cup lime juice
1 cup orange juice
4 tablespoons honey
¼ teaspoon allspice
¼ teaspoon dried thyme
¼ teaspoon cayenne

1 pound tuna steak, cut into 16 1-inch cubes
¼ teaspoon salt
24 1-inch cubes fresh pineapple
2 peeled, pitted mangos, cut into 24 chunks
2 cups cooked long-grain brown rice

1. Stir the lime juice, orange juice, honey, allspice, thyme, and cayenne together in a small bowl. Marinate the fish in 1 cup of the lime juice mixture in the refrigerator 1 hour. Reserve the remaining marinade.

2. Preheat the broiler.

3. Remove the tuna from the marinade and sprinkle with the salt. Thread a piece of pineapple, a piece of mango, and a piece of tuna onto a skewer. Repeat, and then add another piece of each fruit. Fill 8 skewers.

4. Place the kebobs on a baking sheet coated with cooking spray and brush with the reserved marinade. Broil the kebobs 3 minutes. Turn the kebobs, brush with the reserved marinade, and broil 3 to 4 more minutes, or until the tuna is flaky and no longer translucent.

5. Divide the kebobs and rice among 4 plates.

YIELD: 4 servings

COOK'S NOTE: The kebobs can also be prepared on a grill.

Nutritional Information Per Serving

Calories 360 | Energy Density 1.0 | Carbohydrate 56 g. | Fat 3 g. | Protein 30 g. | Fiber 4 g.

Shrimp Creole

Enjoy the flavors of New Orleans in this impressive, easy-to-prepare main dish.

1 cup sliced celery
1 cup chopped onions
2 teaspoons minced garlic
4 cups canned stewed tomatoes
1 cup Tomato and Fresh Basil Sauce
(page 233)
2 teaspoons chili powder

2 tablespoons Worcestershire sauce
1 tablespoon hot-pepper sauce
1 pound boiled shrimp, shelled and
deveined
2 cups green bell pepper strips,
about 1 pound
3 cups cooked brown rice

1. Cook the celery, onions, and garlic in a large pan coated with cooking spray over medium heat until tender, about 5 minutes.

2. Add the tomatoes, tomato sauce, chili powder, Worcestershire sauce, and hot-pepper sauce and simmer, uncovered, 45 minutes. If tomato mixture becomes thick, stir in up to ½ cup water.

3. Add the shrimp and green pepper strips to the tomato mixture and simmer 5 minutes.

4. Divide the rice among 4 plates and spoon the Shrimp Creole over the rice.

YIELD: 4 servings of 1½ cups Shrimp Creole and ¾ cup brown rice each

Nutritional Information Per Serving

Calories 335 | Energy Density 0.60 | Carbohydrate 60 g. | Fat 2 g. | Protein 19 g. | Fiber 8 g.

Shrimp Fried Rice

The rich taste of the dark sesame oil adds a distinctive flavor to this quick stir-fry meal.

3 teaspoons dark sesame oil
¾ pound small shrimp, shelled and
   deveined
2 teaspoons chopped garlic
2 teaspoons chopped fresh ginger
1 cup peeled, finely chopped carrots
1 cup small broccoli florets
¼ cup chopped scallions
1 cup seeded, chopped red or green bell
   peppers

1 cup frozen peas, thawed
2 cups cooked brown rice
1 tablespoon reduced-sodium soy sauce
1 tablespoon hoisin sauce
Pinch cayenne
1 egg
1 egg white

1. Heat 1 teaspoon oil in a large nonstick skillet or wok over medium-high heat. Add the shrimp, garlic, and ginger and stir-fry 3 minutes, or until the shrimp are pink and opaque. Transfer the shrimp to a plate and cover to keep warm.

2. Add 2 teaspoons oil to the skillet and stir-fry the carrots, broccoli, scallions, bell peppers, and peas 2 minutes.

3. Add the rice, soy sauce, hoisin sauce, cayenne, and shrimp and stir-fry 3 minutes, or until heated through.

4. Combine the egg and egg white in a small bowl. Add the eggs to the skillet and cook, stirring occasionally, until the eggs are set.

YIELD: 4 servings of 1½ cups each

COOK'S NOTE: Substitute 6 ounces of tofu for the shrimp for a vegetarian version.

Nutritional Information Per Serving

Calories 325 | Energy Density 1.1 | Carbohydrate 39 g. | Fat 8 g. | Protein 26 g. | Fiber 6 g.

For a 325-calorie entrée

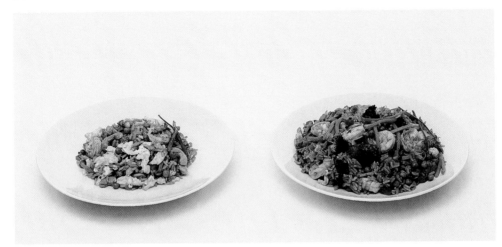

TRADITIONAL	How we lowered the ED	VOLUMETRICS
Stir-fried shrimp with peanuts	▸ Decreased oil ▸ Omitted nuts ▸ Added more vegetables	Shrimp Fried Rice

Fiesta Fish Stew

This low-energy-dense main course will wake up your taste buds with the flavors of the Southwest.

1 cup fish stock or clam juice
1 cup vegetable broth
⅓ cup dry white wine
2 tablespoons lime juice
1 large onion, about 6 ounces, cut into
   ½-inch wedges
2 thinly sliced shallots
1 teaspoon minced garlic
1 seeded, thinly sliced jalapeno

½ teaspoon salt
Pinch freshly ground black pepper
3 cups chopped zucchini
3 seeded finely chopped plum tomatoes
1 pound skinless haddock fillets, cut into
   1¼-inch pieces
2 tablespoons white-wine vinegar
1 cup chopped fresh cilantro

1. Bring the fish stock, broth, wine, lime juice, onions, shallots, garlic, jalapeno, salt, and pepper to a simmer in a 4- to 5-quart saucepan. Cook the mixture, uncovered, 15 minutes.

2. Stir in the zucchini and tomatoes. When the mixture begins to simmer add the haddock and cook 2 minutes, or until the haddock is flaky and no longer translucent. Stir in the vinegar and cilantro. Ladle into 4 soup bowls.

YIELD: 4 servings of 1¾ cups each

COOK'S NOTE: Any white fish fillet such as flounder or sole can be substituted for the haddock.

Nutritional Information Per Serving

Calories 185 | Energy Density 0.40 | Carbohydrate 13 g. | Fat 2 g. | Protein 26 g. | Fiber 3 g.

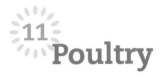

11 Poultry

Poultry can be a dieter's dream. It gives you the protein you need to enhance satiety, and it can be low in energy density. However, eating chicken fried or with the skin can lead to calorie overload. The skin does help to keep the meat juicy while cooking, and very little of the fat from the skin is absorbed during cooking. So, keep the skin on while cooking if you like, just don't eat it. Eating the skin will double the fat grams and add 20 to 40 calories to a 3-ounce serving.

Boneless and skinless cuts of chicken and turkey provide a convenient and versatile source of protein. I use them in several recipes that are quick to prepare and low in calories, such as Chicken Parmesan (page 205) and Italian Turkey Spirals (page 212). Chicken left over from dinner can be part of your lunch the next day. Use it in the Almond Chicken-Salad Sandwich (page 114) or the Thai Chicken Salad (page 142).

Here are more tips on making poultry choices.

- Self-basting whole chickens and turkeys have fat injected into the meat. This extra fat is not necessary for a moist roast—it just adds extra calories.
- Ground poultry can contain the skin, again adding unnecessary fat and calories. Check the label for the lowest fat content, or pick a lean piece of meat and ask to have it ground.
- Make sure when buying frozen precooked chicken, or when ordering chicken in restaurants, that the meat has not been processed and preformed out of various parts, including the skin.
- Dark meat, even without the skin, contains more fat and calories than white

meat. For example, 3 ounces of baked skinless dark chicken meat contains around 150 calories; the same amount of skinless white meat has 120 calories.

- Chicken consumption has increased in recent years and is a popular restaurant item. To make your choice volumetric, order it grilled, baked, or roasted, remove any skin, and surround it with veggies.
- Try making your favorite chicken casserole recipe more volumetric by adding more veggies.

Chicken Parmesan

This is an alternative to traditional fried chicken. It is low in fat, yet high in flavor. Pictured on page 4.

1 teaspoon extra-virgin olive oil
½ teaspoon minced garlic
¼ cup hot-pepper sauce
1 egg white
¼ teaspoon salt

½ cup grated Parmesan cheese
½ cup breadcrumbs (page 175)
¼ cup minced fresh cilantro
4 skinless, boneless chicken breast halves,
   4 to 6 ounces each

1. Preheat the oven to 350 degrees. Lightly coat a baking sheet with cooking spray.

2. In a shallow bowl, whisk the oil, garlic, hot-pepper sauce, egg white, salt, and 2 teaspoons water.

3. In another shallow bowl, combine the Parmesan, breadcrumbs, and cilantro.

4. Dip a chicken breast half in the egg white mixture to coat. Then dredge in the Parmesan mixture to coat completely and place on the baking sheet. Repeat with the remaining chicken. Lightly coat the chicken with cooking spray and bake 35 minutes.

YIELD: 4 servings

COOK'S NOTE: For a different taste, substitute ¼ cup Worcestershire sauce for the hot sauce and chopped, fresh, flat-leaf parsley for the cilantro.

Nutritional Information Per Serving

Calories 200 | Energy Density 1.8 | Carbohydrate 11 g. | Fat 6 g. | Protein 24 g. | Fiber 1 g.

Chicken Merlot

This entrée evokes some of the traditional flavors of French country cooking.

4 skinless, boneless chicken breast halves,
    4 to 6 ounces each
¼ cup all-purpose flour
1 teaspoon dried thyme
½ teaspoon salt
2 teaspoons extra-virgin olive oil
3 cups quartered mushrooms, about ½
    pound

2 cups peeled, sliced carrots
4 pieces Canadian bacon, cut into ¼-inch
    wide slices
⅔ cup Merlot or other dry red wine
⅔ cup nonfat, reduced-sodium chicken
    broth
2 teaspoons tomato paste
¼ cup chopped, fresh, flat-leaf parsley

For a 240-calorie entrée

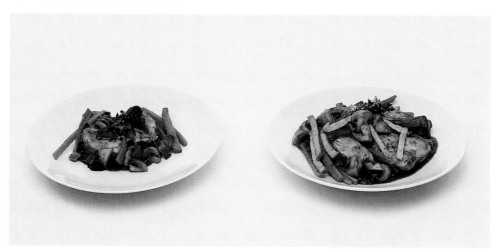

TRADITIONAL	How we lowered the ED	VOLUMETRICS
Coq au vin	▸ Used skinless, white chicken instead of dark meat ▸ Used less oil ▸ Added more veggies ▸ Used Canadian bacon instead of regular bacon	Chicken Merlot

1. Cut each chicken breast crosswise into 3 pieces.

2. Combine the flour, thyme, and salt in a resealable plastic bag and add the chicken pieces. Seal the bag and shake to coat chicken. Remove the chicken and shake off excess flour.

3. Lightly coat a large nonstick skillet with cooking spray. Add 1 teaspoon oil and heat over medium-high heat. Add the chicken and cook, stirring, about 5 minutes, or until the chicken is lightly browned on both sides. Remove the chicken and set it aside.

4. Add 1 teaspoon oil to the skillet and sauté the mushrooms, carrots, and bacon 2 minutes. Stir in the wine, broth, and tomato paste, and cook, stirring occasionally, 10 minutes.

5. Return the chicken to the skillet and cook 4 to 5 minutes, or until it is no longer pink in the center.

6. Divide the chicken mixture among 4 plates, sprinkle with the parsley, and serve.

YIELD: 4 servings

COOK'S NOTE: Try serving the chicken with boiled potatoes, whole-wheat noodles, or short whole-wheat pasta, such as fusilli or penne.

Nutritional Information Per Serving

Calories 240 | Energy Density 0.70 | Carbohydrate 15 g. | Fat 6 g. | Protein 26 g. | Fiber 3 g.

South of the Border Chicken Stew

This zesty dish is a whole meal in one pot.

4 skinless, boneless chicken breast halves,
    4 to 6 ounces each
Salt
Freshly ground black pepper
2 tablespoons extra-virgin olive oil
1½ cups chopped onions
1 cup seeded, chopped green bell peppers
1 cup diced celery
1 teaspoon chopped garlic
2 teaspoons dried oregano

4 cups nonfat, reduced-sodium
    chicken broth
1½ cups frozen corn, thawed
1½ cups canned diced tomatoes, with
    liquid
3 cups baby spinach
¼ teaspoon hot-pepper sauce
½ cup nonfat plain yogurt
¼ cup chopped scallions

1. Cut the chicken into 1-inch chunks and season lightly with salt and pepper.

2. Heat 1 tablespoon of the oil in a 4- to 5-quart pot over medium-high heat. Lightly brown the chicken, stirring, about 5 minutes. Remove the chicken to a bowl.

3. Reduce the heat to medium and add 1 tablespoon oil, onions, bell peppers, celery, and garlic. Cook, stirring frequently, 5 minutes. Stir in the oregano, broth, and ½ teaspoon salt. Bring to a simmer and cook 10 minutes.

4. Stir in the corn, tomatoes, and chicken and simmer 10 minutes, stirring occasionally. Stir in the spinach and hot-pepper sauce.

5. Divide the stew among 4 bowls, and serve with the yogurt and scallions in small bowls on the side.

YIELD: 4 servings of 2½ cups each

Nutritional Information Per Serving

Calories 325 | Energy Density 0.50 | Carbohydrate 24 g. | Fat 11 g. | Protein 34 g. | Fiber 6 g.

For a 325-calorie entrée

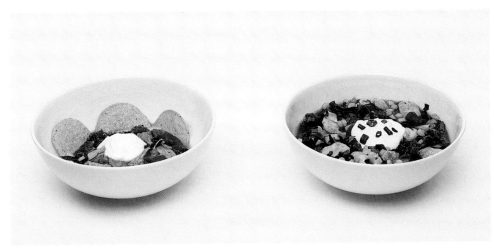

TRADITIONAL	How we lowered the ED	VOLUMETRICS
Mexican stew	▸ Used skinless chicken breast instead of dark meat ▸ Decreased oil ▸ Added more vegetables ▸ Omitted tortilla chips	South of the Border Chicken Stew

Chicken Provençal

Cooking this entrée will fill your kitchen with the aromas of southern French cooking.

1 tablespoon extra-virgin olive oil

4 skinless, boneless chicken breast halves, 4 to 6 ounces each

½ cup chopped onions

1 teaspoon chopped garlic

½ teaspoon salt

Pinch freshly ground black pepper

½ cup dry white wine

1½ cups canned diced tomatoes, with liquid

¼ cup chopped, pitted kalamata or other brine-cured olives

1 tablespoon chopped fresh oregano

1 tablespoon chopped, fresh flat-leaf parsley

1. Heat the oil in a large nonstick skillet over medium heat. Add the chicken, onions, garlic, salt, and pepper. Sautée until the chicken is lightly browned, about 3 minutes on each side.

2. Add the wine and bring to a boil. Add the tomatoes, olives, and oregano and return to the boil. Reduce the heat to low, partially cover, and cook about 6 minutes, or until the chicken is no longer pink.

3. Transfer the chicken to a platter and keep warm. Cook the sauce 2 to 3 minutes, or until it has thickened slightly. Spoon the sauce over the chicken and sprinkle with parsley.

YIELD: 4 servings

COOK'S NOTE: Fresh marjoram is a good substitute for oregano.

Nutritional Information Per Serving

Calories 165 | Energy Density 0.70 | Carbohydrate 7 g. | Fat 5 g. | Protein 18 g. | Fiber 1 g.

Stir-Fried Turkey with Crunchy Vegetables

This quick main-dish uses turkey breast cutlets, a good source of lean protein.

2 teaspoons cornstarch

3 tablespoons soy sauce

1 teaspoon vegetable oil

3 slices fresh ginger, ⅛-inch thick

1 pound turkey breast cutlets, cut into
  ½-inch cubes

1 teaspoon sesame oil

1 cup shredded green cabbage

½ cup sliced onions

1 cup 1-inch-long celery sticks

1 cup 1-inch-long green bell pepper sticks

1 cup 1-inch-long carrot sticks

1 teaspoon chopped garlic

¼ teaspoon freshly ground black pepper

2 cups cooked brown rice

1. Mix the cornstarch with 4 tablespoons cold water in a small bowl to form a thin paste. Stir in the soy sauce and set aside.

2. Heat the vegetable oil in a large, nonstick skillet or wok over high heat. When the oil is hot, add the ginger and stir-fry 1 minute. Remove the ginger with a slotted spoon and discard.

3. Add the turkey to the skillet and stir-fry 3 minutes. Use a slotted spoon to transfer the turkey to a bowl, and set aside.

4. Reduce the heat to medium-high and add the sesame oil. Add the cabbage, onions, celery, bell pepper, carrot, garlic, and black pepper to the skillet and stir-fry 3 minutes.

5. Stir the sauce to recombine and add to the skillet along with the turkey and its juices and stir-fry 2 minutes.

6. Divide the rice and stir-fry mixture among 4 dinner plates.

YIELD: 4 servings of ½ cup rice and ¾ cup stir-fry each

Nutritional Information Per Serving

Calories 330 | Energy Density 0.80 | Carbohydrate 34 g. | Fat 5 g. | Protein 31 g. | Fiber 5 g.

Italian Turkey Spirals

This visually appealing main dish will impress your guests.

1 pound turkey breast cutlets, cut into
   4 equal pieces
4 teaspoons tomato paste
½ cup packed fresh basil leaves
½ teaspoon minced garlic
Salt

Freshly ground black pepper
1 tablespoon nonfat milk
2 tablespoons whole-wheat flour
½ cup Tomato and Fresh Basil Sauce
   (page 233)

1. Set an oven rack about 5 to 6 inches below the broiling element and preheat the broiler.

2. Place the turkey on a work surface and cover with a sheet of plastic wrap. Flatten the turkey to about ¼-inch thick with a meat mallet or rolling pin. Remove the plastic wrap.

3. Spread 1 teaspoon tomato paste on each piece of turkey. Cover with basil leaves, sprinkle on the garlic, and season lightly with salt and pepper.

4. Starting with the short end of the cutlets, roll each piece up tightly and secure with a wooden toothpick. Brush the rolls with milk and lightly dust with flour.

5. Place the rolls on a foil-lined baking sheet and broil, turning occasionally, 20 minutes or until cooked through. Heat the tomato sauce in a small saucepan.

6. Remove the toothpicks and cut each roll, crosswise, into 1-inch-thick pieces. Divide the sliced rolls among 4 plates and spoon 2 tablespoons of the tomato sauce over each. Garnish each with 1 or 2 basil leaves.

YIELD: 4 servings

Nutritional Information Per Serving

Calories 140 | Energy Density 1.0 | Carbohydrate 4 g. | Fat 2 g. | Protein 28 g. | Fiber 1 g.

12 Beans, Rice, and Grains

BEANS AND OTHER LEGUMES

Beans are nutritional powerhouses, rich in protein and fiber as well as vitamins, such as folate. Beans are legumes, which are a family of plants that grow edible seed-bearing pods including peas, beans, lentils, soybeans, and peanuts. One cup of legumes provides about half the daily recommended fiber intake. This can enhance and prolong satiety. For vegetarians, legumes, which include tofu, are an important source of protein.

Most of us are not nearly adventuresome enough with legumes. Look in cookbooks from around the world and you will find that beans and other legumes are used much more widely than in the soups, chili, and baked bean dishes that we are accustomed to eating. I have included recipes that will give you a variety of ways to incorporate legumes into recipes such as Bayou Beans and Rice (page 218) and Chickpea Curry (page 174). Here are some more ideas.

- Use any mashed legume as a meat extender in dishes such as meat loaf or spaghetti sauce.
- Sauté onion, bell pepper, and a mix of legumes together to make a nutritious pilaf.
- Add black beans to Mexican dishes such as tacos and tortillas.
- Sneak beans or split peas into stews and other mixed dishes.

- Include beans or peas in your salads to enhance the fiber, such as in the Tuna and White Bean Salad (page 150).
- Substitute tofu for meat, poultry, or fish in stews, soups, and stir-fries. Try Tofu Pad Thai (page 167)—it is yummy.

You can use canned beans. They are convenient and most of the nutrients remain intact. Make sure you rinse and drain them thoroughly. This helps to remove the added salt and will reduce the compounds that may give you gas.

Speaking of gas, if you are shifting to a higher-fiber diet that includes more legumes and whole grains, you need to make the change slowly. Studies show if you add about 5 grams more daily over a week, your body will adapt. So, if you are eating 15 grams per day now, go up to 20 per day for a week, and then 5 more grams per day the next week until you reach your goal of about 30 to 35 grams per day.

RICE

Rice is one of the most important foods in the human diet. It supplies 20 percent of the calories consumed around the world, and in some Asian countries it contributes more than half the calories consumed. Over 40,000 varieties of rice can be found worldwide. Despite this variety, most of us choose plain long-grain white rice because it is easy to cook, and because the bland taste makes it a versatile addition to many dishes, but white rice has been stripped of the nutrient-rich bran outer layers. Brown rice retains these layers so it is higher in nutrients and fiber, and it is lower in energy density than white rice (1.1 calories per gram compared to 1.3). Brown rice has a chewy texture and a nutty taste, so it does not fit in every recipe. The rice found in your supermarket can be divided into three main types.

- **Long-grain rice** has a long, slender kernel and includes basmati and jasmine rice. Cooked grains are separate (not sticky), light, and fluffy. It is not recommended for cold salads or puddings, since it hardens when cooled.
- **Medium-grain rice** has a shorter, wider kernel than long-grain rice, and it is stickier when cooked. It is often used in recipes that have a creamy consistency such as puddings, and it can be used in salads.

- **Short-grain rice** has a short, almost round kernel. When cooked it is soft and sticky, and you will find it in traditional Chinese cooking and sushi.

GRAINS

You have already heard that you should look for whole grains in breakfast cereals and breads, and that brown, whole-grain rice has more nutrients and fiber than white rice. Let me remind you why you are looking for whole grains. Much of the recent controversy over the amount of carbohydrates we are eating stems from the fact that many of us are eating most of our calories from highly processed, refined carbohydrates—sugars and starches. We should be eating our carbohydrates primarily as whole grains. Instead of seeking our carbohydrates from cookies, cakes, and soda, we should find more nutrient-rich sources. In addition to looking for whole grains in cereals and bread, here are some foods you may not have thought about.

- Corn, even popcorn, counts as whole grain, but foods made from corn meal such as tortillas don't—the processing has removed some of the bran.
- Bulgur is made from wheat kernels that have been steamed, dried, and crushed into small pieces. It has a nutty flavor and a crunchy texture, and cooks quickly. Try Bulgur and Vegetable Stuffed Peppers (page 172).
- Other interesting whole grains to try are barley, buckwheat groats or kasha, millet, and quinoa. Follow package directions to make side dishes or add them to soups and stews. Mary's Quinoa with Lime (page 224) is a tasty, easy-to-prepare side dish.

Garden Chili

This volumetric version of traditional chili has visual appeal and a lower energy density.

1 pound 95 percent lean ground beef

2 cups chopped onions

3 tablespoons chopped garlic

1 cup seeded, chopped green bell peppers

¾ teaspoon salt

¼ teaspoon freshly ground black pepper

3 tablespoons chili powder

2 teaspoons cumin

3 cups canned crushed tomatoes

3 cups nonfat, reduced-sodium beef broth

3 cups canned dark-red kidney beans, rinsed and drained

1 cup chopped celery

2 cup peeled, shredded carrots

1 cup chopped zucchini

1 tablespoon hot-pepper sauce

1. Lightly coat a 4- to 5-quart pot with cooking spray. Heat the pot over medium-high heat until hot. Crumble the beef into the pot and add the onions, garlic, bell peppers, salt, and pepper. Cook, stirring occasionally, until the beef loses its raw color. Drain the liquid from the pot.

2. Reduce the heat to medium and stir in the chili powder and cumin. Add the remaining ingredients and 1 cup water, and bring to a boil, stirring. Cover the pot, reduce the heat, and simmer 45 minutes, stirring occasionally.

YIELD: 8 servings of 1¾ cups each

COOK'S NOTE: Leftover chili is great as a topping for a baked potato.

Nutritional Information Per Serving

Calories 315 | Energy Density 0.70 | Carbohydrate 31 g. | Fat 11 g. | Protein 25 g. | Fiber 11 g.

For a 315-calorie entrée

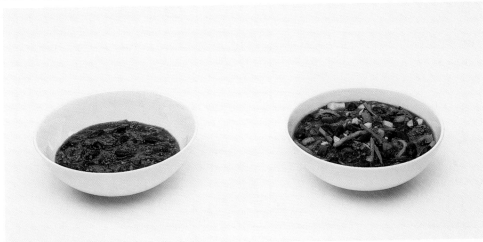

TRADITIONAL	How we lowered the ED	VOLUMETRICS
Beef chili	▸ Used lean ground beef and no oil ▸ Added more veggies	Garden Chili

Bayou Red Beans and Rice

This main dish tastes like the traditional spicy southern staple, but has almost no fat. Keep this recipe in mind for those evenings when you want to get dinner on the table quickly.

1 cup chopped onions

1 teaspoon minced garlic

4 cups canned red kidney beans, rinsed
   and drained

1 cup seeded, diced red bell peppers

1 cup seeded, diced green bell peppers

2 teaspoons cumin

1½ teaspoons hot-pepper sauce

2 cups cooked brown rice

1. Lightly coat a large nonstick skillet with cooking spray and heat over medium-high heat. Add the onions and garlic, and cook, stirring, 5 minutes.

2. Stir in the beans, bell peppers, cumin, hot-pepper sauce, and ½ cup water. Bring to a simmer, cover, and cook 20 minutes.

3. Serve the beans over the rice.

YIELD: 4 servings of 1½ cups each

COOK'S NOTE: The beans and rice can be garnished with chopped scallions. White rice is traditional, but brown has more fiber and nutrients.

Nutritional Information Per Serving

Calories. 300 | Energy Density 0.90 | Carbohydrate 60 g. | Fat 1 g. | Protein 14 g. | Fiber 15 g.

For a 300-calorie entrée

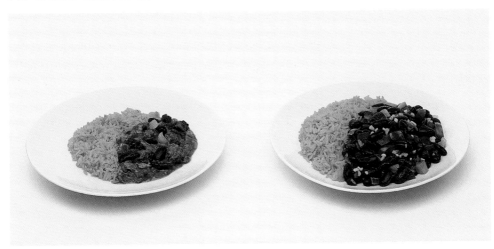

TRADITIONAL	How we lowered the ED	VOLUMETRICS
Red beans and rice with ham	▸ Omitted high-fat meat, oil, and lard ▸ Added peppers and more onion	Bayou Beans and Rice

Paella Sencillo

This simplified version of the classic Spanish rice dish is delicious and ready to serve in under an hour.

¼ pound turkey kielbasa

1 tablespoon vegetable oil

¼ pound skinless, boneless chicken breast, cut into ½-inch cubes

½ cup chopped onions

¾ cup long-grain rice

1 teaspoon chopped garlic

¼ teaspoon crushed saffron threads or ¼ teaspoon turmeric

1¼ cups nonfat, reduced-sodium, chicken broth

¾ cup fish stock or clam juice

¼ teaspoon salt

¼ teaspoon freshly ground black pepper

1 cup frozen baby peas, thawed

¼ pound medium shrimp, shelled and deveined

4 lemon wedges

1. Preheat the broiler.

2. Broil the kielbasa for 7 minutes on each side. Slice it in half lengthwise, cut across into ½-inch-thick pieces, and set aside.

3. Lightly spray a large skillet or paella pan with cooking spray. Add 1 teaspoon oil and heat over medium heat. Add the chicken and cook, stirring, 7 minutes. Remove the chicken with a slotted spoon to a bowl and set aside.

4. Add 2 teaspoons oil, onions, rice, and garlic to the skillet. Cook 4 minutes, stirring often. Stir the saffron into the broth and add to the skillet. Add the stock, salt, and pepper and simmer 30 minutes, covered.

5. Stir in the kielbasa, chicken, peas, and shrimp. Cook the paella, covered, 5 minutes, or until the shrimp are done. Serve the paella garnished with lemon wedges.

YIELD: 4 servings of 1¼ cups each

Nutritional Information Per Serving

Calories 325 | Energy Density 1.2 | Carbohydrate 41 g. | Fat 8 g. | Protein 27 g. | Fiber 3 g.

Vegetable Pilaf

In a pilaf, rice is sautéed in butter or oil before adding the liquid. The energy density of this side dish has been lowered by adding vegetables to simmer along with the rice.

2 teaspoons unsalted butter
½ cup chopped onions
½ cup long-grain white rice
½ cup vegetable broth
½ cup trimmed, diced, thin asparagus
½ cup chopped mushrooms,
   about 2 ounces

¼ teaspoon dried tarragon
¼ teaspoon salt
½ cup diced zucchini
½ cup frozen baby peas, thawed

1. Melt the butter in a 4- to 5-quart saucepan over medium heat. Add the onions and cook 3 minutes. Add the rice and stir to coat in the butter.

2. Stir in ½ cup water, broth, asparagus, mushrooms, tarragon, and salt and bring to a simmer. Cover and cook over low heat 16 to 20 minutes, or until the rice is tender and all the liquid has been absorbed.

3. Fold the zucchini and peas into the rice. Cover, and let stand, 3 minutes.

YIELD: 4 servings of ¾ cup each

Nutritional Information Per Serving

Calories 135 | Energy density 0.90 | Carbohydrate 25 g. | Fat 2 g. | Protein 4 g. | Fiber 2 g.

Risotto Primavera

This main dish is a delicious low-fat version of traditional risotto.

1½ cups vegetable broth
1 tablespoon extra-virgin olive oil
1 cup chopped onions
1 cup trimmed, diced fresh green beans
1 cup seeded, chopped red bell peppers
1 cup peeled, diced carrots
1 tablespoon plus ¼ cup chopped fresh basil

1 teaspoon chopped garlic
1 cup short-grain rice
½ cup dry white wine
1 tablespoon grated Parmesan cheese
Freshly ground black pepper

1. Bring the broth and 1½ cups water to a simmer in a saucepan. Keep warm over low heat.

2. Heat the oil in a 4- to 5-quart nonstick pot over medium-high heat. Add the onions, beans, bell peppers, carrots, 1 tablespoon basil, and garlic and cook, stirring, 6 minutes.

3. Add the rice and cook, stirring constantly, 2 minutes.

4 Add the wine and 1 cup of broth and cook, stirring constantly, until the liquid is nearly absorbed. Add the remaining broth, ½ cup at a time, stirring often, until liquid is absorbed before adding the next portion, about 25 to 30 minutes total cooking time.

5. Remove the risotto from the heat and stir in the Parmesan and a few grindings of black pepper.

6. Divide among 4 plates garnished with the remaining basil.

YIELD: 4 servings of 1½ cups each

COOK'S NOTE: The wine can be replaced by vegetable broth. Although Arborio or Italian rice is usually specified for risotto, any short-grain rice will give excellent results. Risotto may be made ahead and held for up to an hour. To do that, reserve 1 cup of the broth. Stop the process when the remaining broth is used up. Take the risotto off the heat, cover, and set aside. When ready to proceed, uncover and reheat slowly over medium heat, stirring, being careful not to burn it. Increase the heat to medium-high, add the reserved broth ½ cup at a time, and the rest of the ingredients as directed.

Nutritional Information Per Serving

Calories 290 | Energy Density 1.0 | Carbohydrate 51 g. | Fat 5 g. | Protein 6 g. | Fiber 5 g.

For a 290-calorie entrée

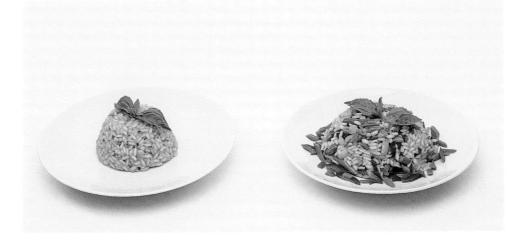

TRADITIONAL	How we lowered the ED	VOLUMETRICS
Risotto	▸ Decreased butter and cheese ▸ Added vegetables	Risotto Primavera

Mary's Quinoa with Lime

Quinoa is a grain with a delicious nutty flavor that has been cultivated in South America for centuries. Serve this light and refreshing recipe as a side dish. Mary is a friend and colleague of mine who is always willing to share her favorite volumetric recipes.

4 tablespoons lime juice

1 tablespoon extra-virgin olive oil

1 tablespoon plus 1 cup vegetable broth

1 tablespoon seeded, finely chopped jalapeno

3 tablespoons chopped fresh cilantro

½ teaspoon sugar

¼ teaspoon salt

⅛ teaspoon freshly ground black pepper

½ cup quinoa

1 teaspoon toasted cumin seeds (page 84)

1 cup canned black beans, rinsed and drained

1 cup seeded, chopped orange bell peppers

1 cup seeded, chopped red bell peppers

3 tablespoons chopped scallions

1. In a medium bowl, whisk together the lime juice, oil, 1 tablespoon broth, jalapeno, cilantro, sugar, salt, and pepper. Set aside.

2. Bring 1 cup broth to a boil in a small saucepan. Add the quinoa and cumin seed. Simmer, covered, 10 minutes, or until the broth is absorbed.

3. Combine the black beans, bell peppers, and scallions in a large bowl. Fluff the quinoa with a fork and add to the bowl. Toss the mixture with the lime dressing and chill 1 hour.

YIELD: 4 servings of ¾ cup each

COOK'S NOTE: Quinoa can be found in the international section of large supermarkets, some health-food stores, and some specialty grocery stores.

Nutritional Information Per Serving

Calories 195 | Energy Density 0.77 | Carbohydrate 32 g. | Fat 5 g. | Protein 7 g. | Fiber 6 g.

13 Pasta and Pizza

Two of America's most popular foods, pasta and pizza, are consumed by millions of us each day. Italians shudder when they see how we eat these foods. It is our usual problem—we are eating too much. Our portions are huge, and we have added fat and calories that we don't need. Despite what you hear from advocates of low-carbohydrate diets, it makes no sense to avoid pasta and pizza. They are too good, too convenient, and too nutritious to give up. Instead I will show you how to fit them in to your healthy *Volumetrics Eating Plan*.

PASTA

In my lab, we have used pasta dishes in a number of our satiety studies. We have shown that the bigger the portion of macaroni and cheese or baked ziti we served, the more people ate—and most did not notice that the portions were bigger. Other studies in my lab have shown how to manage calories even when served large portions. The answer won't surprise you: Reduce the energy density by increasing the vegetables in your pasta dishes and decreasing the fat. When given unlimited amounts, the people in our studies served themselves the same amount of our pasta dishes. Thus, when we reduced the energy density by adding vegetables, they consumed fewer calories, and they were just as full and satisfied.

Another way to boost satiety is to look for whole-grain pasta. It is chewier and has a more distinct taste than regular pasta, but it is worth trying because you can get 5 to 6 grams of fiber in each serving. Or you can try wheat-blended pasta; it is similar to regular pasta and contains 3 grams of fiber. Regular pasta is made with processed wheat flour that contains little fiber. Some pasta has added soy flour that boosts the protein content.

Pasta is one of the most versatile ingredients in our culinary repertoire. Here are some tips on how to prepare healthy pasta dishes.

- Be creative. Just about any combination of vegetables can be used to top pasta. Sauté olive oil, garlic, tomatoes, and other vegetables such as zucchini, yellow squash, asparagus, mushrooms, or eggplant, and toss with cooked pasta.
- Keep your favorite fresh herbs available. Basil, with its distinctive flavor, is a favorite. Or try cilantro for a south-of-the-border twist.
- When in a hurry, you can use bottled sauce, but be sure to check the fat content, as it can vary widely.
- Experiment with different pasta shapes. Instead of traditional spaghetti, try linguine, farfalle, fettuccine, penne, or angel-hair pasta.
- For a high-satiety meal, add protein to the sauce. Legumes such as beans or lentils add variety and texture, or you can use fish, ground turkey breast, and lean chicken or beef. Oceanside Pasta is a delicious combination of pasta and shellfish (page 230).
- Be aware of appropriate portions. A serving of cooked pasta is only one-half cup, which contains about 100 calories. You can eat more, but your best strategy is to limit the pasta you eat at a meal to one cup and to bulk up the meal with vegetables and lean protein.

PIZZA

You can eat pizza when managing your weight—I will show you how and give you several delicious recipes. There are many ways to make pizza, and it is simple to adjust the proportions of the various ingredients to reduce calories and enhance satiety. For example, in the pizza recipes, using packaged wheat pizza dough and stretching it thin saved 100 calories per slice compared to a packaged white-flour crust. Here are some more tips on how to make your own nutritious pizza.

- Fun and quick individual pizzas can be made with whole-wheat pita bread or English muffins instead of pizza crust.
- To cut down on total fat and saturated fat use nonfat or reduced-fat mozzarella and cut back on the amount of cheese you usually use.

- Try using grated Parmesan cheese as a topping. Its intense flavor means you only need a small amount.
- For a low-fat white pizza (without tomato sauce) such as The Aristotle Pizza (page 237), use reduced-fat ricotta cheese.
- Be generous with the veggie toppings. Add fresh chopped tomato, onion, artichokes, roasted red peppers, broccoli, zucchini, or mushrooms. Experiment with new combinations such as those in the Garden Fresh Vegetable Pizza (page 238).
- As when preparing pasta, it is good to have fresh herbs such as oregano, marjoram, thyme, or basil on hand.
- Give the pizza some bite with hot peppers—this helps ensure that you won't notice that the fat has been reduced.
- Enhance satiety by adding lean protein: Try seafood, such as shrimp or clams; poultry; reduced-fat sausage; tofu; or beans.
- If you want pepperoni on your pizza, give Turkey-Pepperoni Pizza (page 242) a try.
- Pizza doesn't have to be Italian. Chicken Fajita Pizza (page 240) will give you a taste of Mexico.

I am sure you don't always want to make your own pizza. If you know how to choose, pizza can be a reasonable option when eating out. Some pizza chains are making it easy by adding healthy selections to their menus. If these are not available, here are some pizza strategies.

- Much of the fat and calories comes from the cheese. If the pizza is made to order, you can request less cheese. If the cheese is already there, you don't have to eat it all! You can also soak up some of the fat from the top of the pizza with a napkin.
- Instead of pepperoni or sausage, go for lower-fat meat options, such as chicken, Canadian bacon, or ham. Skip the meat if no low-fat options are available.
- You can save calories by ordering a thin-crust pizza.
- Top your pizza with lots of vegetables. Ask if vegetables can be substituted for some of the cheese.
- Know how many calories there are per slice. Many chain restaurants have this information on their websites. I checked out several and found the size of a slice varies a lot and so does the calorie count—from 140 to 500 calories per slice!
- Eat a salad before, or along with, your pizza. This is one way to eat only one slice of pizza, but still feel satisfied.

Charlie's Pasta Primavera

There are lots of combinations of vegetables that work with pasta. Charlie has tried many, but this is his favorite. It is delicious without the usual butter or cream.

1 tablespoon extra-virgin olive oil
1 cup seeded, chopped bell peppers of
  any color
1 cup chopped onions
1 teaspoon chopped garlic
2 cups diced zucchini
1 pound thin asparagus, trimmed and
  cut into 1-inch lengths

2 cups cored, chopped fresh tomatoes
2 tablespoons fresh oregano
1 teaspoon salt
Pinch freshly ground black pepper
8 ounces dry whole-wheat penne
4 cups baby spinach
4 tablespoons grated Parmesan cheese

For a 345-calorie entrée

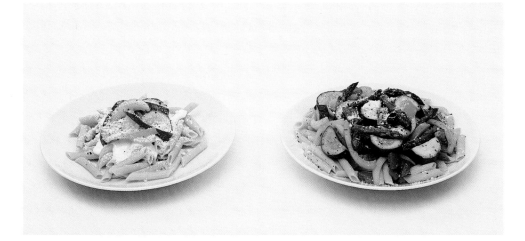

TRADITIONAL	How we lowered the ED	VOLUMETRICS
Pasta primavera	▸ Decreased the amount of pasta ▸ Increased the amount of veggies ▸ Omitted cream sauce	Charlie's Pasta Primavera

1. Heat the oil in a large nonstick skillet over medium heat. Add the bell peppers, onions, and garlic and cook, stirring frequently, 5 minutes.

2. Add the zucchini, asparagus, tomatoes, oregano, salt, and pepper. Stir well. Reduce the heat to medium-low and cook, uncovered, 10 to 15 minutes, stirring occasionally. Keep the sauce warm over low heat.

3. Cook the penne as directed on the package. Reserve ½ cup cooking water and drain the pasta.

4. Add the penne and spinach to the sauce and stir thoroughly. Let the mixture sit over low heat about 1 minute.

5. Stir in about ¼ cup reserved cooking water. Add more if the mixture looks dry.

6. Divide the pasta among 4 dinner plates or shallow bowls and sprinkle with Parmesan.

YIELD: 4 servings of 3 cups each

COOK'S NOTE: Any medium whole-wheat pasta can be substituted for the penne, such as zitti, rotelle, or farfalle. Fresh green beans cut into 1-inch lengths can be substituted for the asparagus.

Nutritional Information Per Serving

Calories 345 | Energy Density 0.80 | Carbohydrate 59 g. | Fat 7 g. | Protein 15 g. | Fiber 10 g.

Oceanside Pasta

Shellfish combine beautifully with tomatoes and pasta in this delicious and satisfying main course.

½ pound unshelled medium shrimp
½ pound sea scallops
1 tablespoon extra-virgin olive oil
1 large garlic clove, peeled and cut in half
½ cup chopped onions
3½ cups canned chopped tomatoes, with liquid
½ teaspoon salt

Freshly ground black pepper
½ teaspoon dried oregano
¼ teaspoon crushed red-pepper flakes
8 ounces dry, medium, whole-wheat pasta shells
1 teaspoon grated lemon zest
2 tablespoons lemon juice
3 tablespoons chopped fresh basil

1. Bring 6 cups water to a boil in a medium saucepan. Add the shrimp and cook 2 to 3 minutes, or until the shrimp turn pink. Drain the shrimp and cool. Shell and devein the shrimp, cut each in half lengthwise, and set aside.

2. Cut the scallops in half horizontally and drain in a colander. Dry the scallops with paper towels and set aside.

3. Heat the oil in a large skillet over medium heat. Add the garlic and sauté, pressing on the pieces with a spatula, 2 minutes, or until they turn golden. Remove and discard.

4. Add the onions to the skillet and cook 5 minutes, stirring occasionally.

5. Stir in the tomatoes, salt, a few grindings of black pepper, oregano, and red-pepper flakes. Bring to a simmer and cook 25 minutes.

6. Prepare the pasta shells as directed on the package and drain.

7. Add the shrimp and scallops to the sauce and cook 3 to 5 minutes, or until the scallops turn opaque.

8. Drain the pasta and add it to the sauce along with the zest, lemon juice, and basil. Stir well and serve.

YIELD: 4 servings of 2 cups each

COOK'S NOTE: If you prefer, you can use all scallops or all shrimp.

Nutritional Information Per Serving					
Calories 400	Energy Density 0.80	Carbohydrate 54 g.	Fat 7 g.	Protein 31 g.	Fiber 4 g.

Penne with Olives and Spinach

This tasty entrée features ingredients typically used in Mediterranean cooking.

8 ounces dry, whole-wheat penne or other medium whole-wheat pasta

1 tablespoon extra-virgin olive oil

1 teaspoon red-wine vinegar

1 teaspoon chopped garlic

¼ cup chopped, pitted kalamata or other brine-cured olives

1 tablespoon drained capers, chopped if large

Salt

Freshly ground black pepper

4 cups baby spinach

2 tablespoons grated Parmesan cheese

1. Cook the penne as directed on the package and drain.

2. Whisk the oil, vinegar, garlic, olives, and capers in a large bowl. Season lightly with salt and pepper.

3. Add the spinach, Parmesan, and penne to the bowl and toss well. Serve warm or at room temperature.

YIELD: 4 servings of 1½ cups each

COOK'S NOTE: Arugula can be substituted for the spinach.

Nutritional Information Per Serving

Calories 265 | Energy Density 1.4 | Carbohydrate 43 g. | Fat 6 g. | Protein 9 g. | Fiber 5 g.

Spaghetti with Tomato and Fresh Basil Sauce

This main dish recipe contains a delicious and simply made marinara sauce that is low in calories and fat.

1 teaspoon extra-virgin olive oil

1 cup chopped onions

1½ teaspoons chopped garlic

3½ cups canned crushed tomatoes

½ teaspoon dry oregano

¼ teaspoon crushed red-pepper flakes

1 teaspoon salt

Freshly ground black pepper

1 cup chopped fresh basil

12 ounces dry, whole-wheat spaghetti

4 tablespoons grated Parmesan cheese

1. Lightly coat a large skillet with cooking spray. Heat the skillet with the oil over medium heat. Add the onions and cook 5 minutes, stirring occasionally. Add the garlic, tomatoes, oregano, red-pepper flakes, salt, and a few grindings of black pepper and simmer 15 minutes, stirring occasionally. Reduce the heat to low and stir the basil into the sauce.

2. Cook the spaghetti as directed on the package. Reserve ¼ cup cooking water and drain.

3. Add the spaghetti to the Tomato and Fresh Basil Sauce. Stir to combine and let it sit 1 minute. If the sauce looks dry, stir in the reserved cooking water.

4. Divide the spaghetti among 4 dinner plates and sprinkle with Parmesan.

YIELD: 4 servings of 2 cups each

COOK'S NOTE: If you prefer a smoother sauce, puree it before adding the spaghetti. This recipe produces about 3½ cups of sauce, which can be used in any recipe calling for tomato sauce. It freezes well.

Nutritional Information Per Serving

Calories 400 | Energy Density 1.0 | Carbohydrate 80 g. | Fat 5 g. | Protein 15 g. | Fiber 5 g.

Nutritional Information Per Serving of Tomato Sauce

Calories 100 | Energy Density 0.40 | Carbohydrate 16 g. | Fat 3 g. | Protein 4 g. | Fiber 3 g.

Veggie-Stuffed Macaroni and Cheese

This volumetric main course shows that you can enjoy the ultimate comfort food while managing your weight.

8 ounces dry, whole-wheat elbow macaroni, fusilli, or penne
2 tablespoons whole-wheat breadcrumbs (page 175)
1 teaspoon melted butter
¼ teaspoon paprika
1¾ cups nonfat milk
3 tablespoons all-purpose flour
2 cups shredded, reduced-fat Cheddar cheese

1 cup 1 percent fat cottage cheese
¼ cup grated Parmesan cheese
Pinch grated nutmeg
½ teaspoon salt
Pinch freshly ground black pepper
6 cups shredded fresh spinach, about 1 pound
1½ cups canned diced tomatoes, with liquid

1. Preheat the oven to 375 degrees.

2. Lightly coat a 9-by-13-inch baking dish with cooking spray.

3. Cook the pasta according to the package directions. Drain and set aside.

4. Mix the breadcrumbs, butter, and paprika in a small bowl and set aside.

5. Heat 1½ cups milk in a 4- to 5-quart nonstick saucepan over medium-high heat until steaming.

6. Whisk the remaining ¼ cup milk and the flour in a small bowl until smooth. Add to the hot milk and cook, whisking constantly, until the sauce thickens and simmers, 3 to 7 minutes. Remove the pan from the heat.

7. Add the Cheddar to the white sauce and stir until the cheese is melted. Stir in the cottage cheese, Parmesan, nutmeg, salt, and pepper. Stir the pasta into the cheese sauce.

8. Spread half of the pasta mixture into the baking dish. Place the spinach evenly on

top, then the diced tomatoes. Spread the remaining pasta mixture over the tomatoes and sprinkle with the breadcrumb mixture.

9. Bake until bubbly and golden, 25 to 30 minutes.

YIELD: 6 servings of 1½ cups each

COOK'S NOTE: Two cups chopped fresh broccoli florets can be substituted for the spinach.

Nutritional Information Per Serving

Calories 330 | Energy Density 1.0 | Carbohydrate 38 g. | Fat 9 g. | Protein 25 g. | Fiber 5 g.

For a 330-calorie entrée

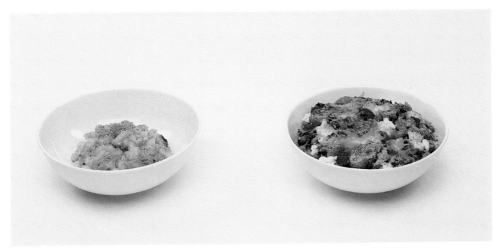

TRADITIONAL	How we lowered the ED	VOLUMETRICS
Macaroni and cheese	▸ Used whole-wheat pasta, nonfat milk, and reduced-fat cheese ▸ Reduced the amount of butter and cheese ▸ Added vegetables	Veggie-Stuffed Macaroni and Cheese

Broccoli and Tomato Stuffed Shells

Baked stuffed pasta shells are a familiar Italian entrée. Here, using less cheese and adding broccoli and tomatoes to the stuffing lowers the energy density.

20 dry jumbo pasta shells
1 cup 1 percent fat cottage cheese
¾ cup shredded, part-skim mozzarella
  cheese
¼ cup grated Parmesan cheese
1 egg
½ teaspoon minced garlic

½ teaspoon freshly ground black pepper
1 cup chopped fresh broccoli florets
1½ cups canned diced tomatoes,
  with liquid
⅓ cup chopped fresh basil
2 cups Tomato and Fresh Basil Sauce
  (page 233)

1. Preheat the oven to 375 degrees.

2. Cook the pasta shells according to the package directions. Drain and set aside.

3. Combine the cottage cheese, mozzarella, Parmesan, egg, garlic, and black pepper in a large bowl and mix well. Add the broccoli, tomatoes, and basil and mix gently.

4. Spread ½ cup tomato sauce on the bottom of a 9-by-13-inch glass baking dish.

5. Put 2 tablespoons of the cheese mixture into each shell. Place the shells in the dish. Gently cover the shells with the remaining 1½ cups tomato sauce.

6. Cover the dish with foil and bake 45 minutes.

YIELD: 4 servings of 5 shells each

COOK'S NOTE: Chopped frozen spinach can be substituted for the broccoli. Thaw and squeeze out the excess liquid.

Nutritional Information Per Serving

Calories 370 | Energy Density 1 | Carbohydrate 47 g. | Fat 9 g. | Protein 25 g. | Fiber 5 g.

The Aristotle Pizza

Feta cheese and fresh dill add great flavor to this colorful, Greek-inspired, vegetarian pizza.

9 ounces packaged wheat pizza dough
  (see Cook's Note)
1 cup nonfat ricotta cheese
1 teaspoon extra-virgin olive oil
1 teaspoon chopped garlic
1 cup chopped onions

3 cups shredded fresh spinach
5 plum tomatoes cut into ¼-inch-thick
  slices
½ cup nonfat feta cheese
1 tablespoon chopped fresh dill

1. Preheat the oven to 375 degrees.

2. Stretch the dough out on a 12-inch pizza pan or roll out into a 12-inch round on a baking sheet.

3. Spread the ricotta evenly over the dough, leaving a ¼-inch border.

4. Heat the oil over medium-high heat in a large skillet coated with cooking spray. Add the garlic, onions, and spinach and sauté, stirring frequently, 5 minutes.

5. Spread the spinach mixture over the ricotta. Cover with the tomato slices and feta. Sprinkle with dill.

6. Bake until the crust is golden, 20 to 25 minutes. Cut the pizza into 4 wedges.

YIELD: 4 servings

COOK'S NOTE: Packaged wheat pizza dough made with whole-wheat flour is available in larger supermarkets. If packaged pizza dough is not available at your local store, a pre-made crust can be used, but it will increase the calorie level by approximately 100 calories per serving.

Nutritional Information Per Serving

Calories 290 | Energy Density 1.0 | Carbohydrate 34 g. | Fat 6 g. | Protein 21 g. | Fiber 5 g.

Garden-Fresh Vegetable Pizza

This recipe makes an eye-catching pizza. The vegetables complement the traditional tomatoes and mozzarella.

1 tablespoon extra-virgin olive oil

1 cup thinly sliced leeks, white part only

1 teaspoon minced garlic

1 cup peeled, grated carrots

9 ounces packaged wheat pizza dough (page 237)

2 medium tomatoes, cored and cut into ¼-inch slices

½ cup thinly sliced zucchini

1 cup thin asparagus, cut into 1-inch-long pieces

Salt

Freshly ground black pepper

½ cup shredded, nonfat mozzarella cheese

1. Preheat the oven to 375 degrees.

2. Heat the oil in a nonstick skillet over medium heat. Add the leeks and garlic and cook, stirring occasionally, 4 minutes. Stir in the carrots and cook 1 minute. Remove the skillet from the heat and set aside.

3. Stretch the dough out in a 12-inch pizza pan or roll out into a 12-inch round on a baking sheet.

4. Spread the leek mixture onto the dough, leaving a ½-inch border.

5. Arrange the tomato slices around the outside edge of the leek mixture and lay the zucchini slices in the center. Place the asparagus on top of the tomatoes. Season lightly with the salt and pepper. Sprinkle the mozzarella over the pizza.

6. Bake until the crust is golden, about 15 to 20 minutes. Cut the pizza into 4 wedges.

YIELD: 4 servings.

Nutritional Information Per Serving

Calories 285 | Energy Density 1.2 | Carbohydrate 41 g. | Fat 9 g. | Protein 13 g. | Fiber 5 g.

Pizza Margherita

This is a lower fat version of a Neapolitan favorite.

9 ounces packaged wheat pizza dough
    (page 237)
5 plum tomatoes, thinly sliced
½ teaspoon minced garlic

⅛ teaspoon salt
Pinch freshly ground black pepper
1 cup shredded, nonfat mozzarella cheese
½ cup chopped fresh basil

1. Preheat the oven to 375 degrees.

2. Stretch the dough out in a 12-inch pizza pan or roll out into a 12-inch round on a baking sheet.

3. Arrange the tomatoes on the dough in overlapping slices, leaving a ½-inch border. Sprinkle evenly with the garlic, salt, black pepper, and mozzarella. Bake for 15 to 20 minutes or until the crust is golden brown. Sprinkle with the basil and cut into 4 wedges.

YIELD: 4 servings

Nutritional Information Per Serving

Calories 265 | Energy Density 1.3 | Carbohydrate 37 g. | Fat 7 g. | Protein 16 g. | Fiber 4 g.

Chicken Fajita Pizza

This unusual pizza has the flavors of Mexican cooking.

5 cherry tomatoes

2 tablespoons chopped cilantro

2 tablespoons chopped onions

1½ teaspoons seeded and finely chopped
  jalapeno pepper

1½ teaspoons lime juice

Dash salt

2 tablespoons reduced-fat sour cream

2 cups seeded, diced bell peppers, any color

½ cup diced red onions

1 cup diced cooked chicken breast
  (page 114)

⅓ cup canned black beans, rinsed and
  drained

½ cup cored, diced red tomatoes

2 teaspoons ground cumin

2 teaspoons chili powder

9 ounces packaged wheat pizza dough
  (page 237)

1 cup shredded, low-fat Cheddar cheese

1. Preheat the oven to 375 degrees.

2. Combine the tomatoes, cilantro, onions, jalapeno, juice, and salt in a small bowl. Set the Cherry Tomato Salsa aside.

3. Combine ¼ cup of the salsa and sour cream in a small bowl and set aside.

4. Heat a medium-sized skillet over medium heat. Add the bell peppers, onions, chicken, beans, tomatoes, cumin, and chili powder to the skillet and cook for 2 to 3 minutes, just long enough to soften the vegetables slightly. Remove the skillet from the heat and set it aside.

5. Stretch the dough out in a 12-inch pizza pan or roll out into a 12-inch round on a baking sheet.

6. Spread the salsa mixture evenly over the dough leaving a ½-inch border.

7. Spread the Cheddar evenly over the salsa mixture. Follow with the bell pepper mixture.

8. Bake for 15 to 20 minutes or until the crust is golden brown. Cut the pizza into 4 wedges.

YIELD: 4 servings

COOK'S NOTE: Use the Cherry Tomato Salsa as a dip with raw vegetables or as a topping for baked potatoes.

Nutritional Information Per Serving

Calories 390 | Energy Density 1.6 | Carbohydrate 41 g. | Fat 15 g. | Protein 24 g. | Fiber 5 g.

Nutritional Information Per 2 Tablespoon Serving of Salsa

Calories 10 | Energy Density 0.25 | Carbohydrate 3 g. | Fat 1 g. | Protein 1 g. | Fiber 1 g.

For a 390-calorie pizza entrée

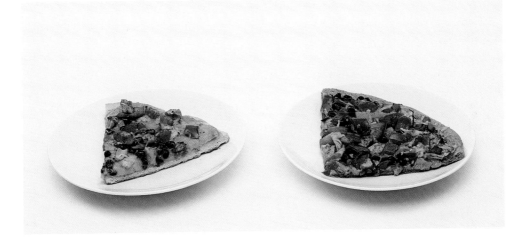

TRADITIONAL	How we lowered the ED	VOLUMETRICS
Chicken topped pizza	▸ Used less dough and cheese ▸ Used whole-wheat dough, and reduced-fat sour cream and cheese ▸ Increased the amount of veggies	Chicken Fajita Pizza

Turkey-Pepperoni Pizza

Using turkey pepperoni reduces the calories and fat, while retaining the same spicy flavor of traditional pepperoni pizza.

1 green bell pepper, cut into strips
½ cup sliced red onions
¾ cup sliced mushrooms, about 3 ounces
9 ounces packaged wheat pizza dough (page 237)

½ cup prepared low-fat pizza sauce
1 cup shredded, 2 percent fat mozzarella cheese
1 ounce turkey pepperoni, cut into about 16 slices, each the size of a fifty-cent piece

1. Preheat oven to 375 degrees.

2. Spray a nonstick skillet with cooking spray. Heat the skillet over medium heat and add the bell peppers, onions, and mushrooms. Sauté until the vegetables are slightly tender, about 4 to 5 minutes. Remove the skillet from the heat and set aside.

3. Stretch the dough out in a 12-inch pizza pan or roll out into a 12-inch round on a baking sheet.

4. Spread the pizza sauce on the dough, leaving a ½-inch border.

5. Spread the mozzarella evenly over the pizza sauce. Cover with the pepperoni and vegetable mixture.

6. Bake the pizza 15 to 20 minutes, or until the crust is golden brown. Cut the pizza into 4 wedges.

YIELD: 4 servings

Nutritional Information Per Serving

Calories 295 | Energy Density 1.6 | Carbohydrate 36 g. | Fat 10 g. | Protein 18 g. | Fiber 3 g.

Desserts and Fruit

Why do we always have room for dessert? Satiety can be food specific, so that although you have had enough of your entrée, foods with different tastes or textures can still taste as good as they did at the start of the meal. This *sensory-specific satiety* explains why you still enjoy the sweet taste of dessert after eating your fill of salty or savory foods earlier in the meal. It also explains why you can keep eating after you have satisfied your body's need for food. Dessert can be enormously pleasurable and, for some of us, a meal may not feel complete without it. However, if you find in your food diary that you are eating a big portion of your daily calories at dessert, you need to develop strategies that keep dessert calories in check without leaving you feeling deprived.

It is not dessert that is the problem, but what and how much you are eating. It is okay to eat high-calorie, energy-dense desserts as a special treat, but remember that you need to exert portion control. For many of us, we are more likely to eat this type of dessert when we are out with friends. In one study, we found that groups of friends ate 50 percent more calories at a meal together than when they ate alone or with strangers. Almost all of the extra calories came from dessert. The obvious strategy is to share dessert. I find this happening more and more, even at business dinners. Restaurants are usually happy to bring extra plates and forks to the table.

If you make your own dessert, there are many ways you can make it a nutritious choice. When baking, explore recipes that use reduced-fat ingredients such as low-fat milk or egg whites instead of whole eggs. Or replace fat with fruit such as applesauce or prunes (now often called dried plums). For added fiber and nutrients, experiment with whole-grain flour by using it to replace a third of the regular flour.

Another option is to choose a low-calorie dessert such as sorbet, or seasonal fruit. Dessert is an ideal time to add more fruit to your day. Like vegetables, most fruits are high in fiber, and their high water content makes them very low in energy density. To ensure that you take advantage of the array of nutrients found in fruits, choose a variety of colors—purple, red, yellow, green, blue, or orange. Fresh fruit is best, especially if it is in season, but frozen fruit with no added sugar or canned fruit in its own juice or water can be substituted when fresh is not available. To get more fiber and boost satiety, leave the skin on when you can.

I know this is a chapter about dessert, and I do give you some chocolate in the Chocolate Fondue with Fresh Fruit (page 259). Indeed, I am an advocate of finishing your meal with a piece of delicious chocolate—doing so can send a signal that you are finished eating and truly satisfied. However, I want to leave you with some thoughts about why you should be eating more fruits—not just for dessert, but whenever you can fit them into your day.

Many fruits are so low in energy density that you don't have to worry about how much you eat. Melon, citrus, and berries provide satisfying portions for few calories. For example, if you are looking for a 100-calorie snack, you get 1¼ cups of orange segments or 2¾ cups of strawberries. Remember, these numbers apply to fruit without added sugar or cream. In this section's recipes, I have chosen some delicious fruit-based desserts that will feel like treats without too many calories. Here are a few more tips on how to add fruit to your day.

- Keep your kitchen stocked with fruits that keep well, such as apples, pears, and citrus fruits. You can pick up more perishable items, like berries, more frequently.
- Add fresh, frozen, or canned fruits to dishes you already like (such as berries or bananas to yogurt).
- Pack bite-sized fruit in lunch bags for school or work: apple slices, grapes, berries, orange quarters, or clementines. Single servings of easy-to-open containers of fruit and applesauce are also convenient.
- Experiment with adding fruit to salad. Try Fennel, Orange, and Arugula Salad (page 133), or Fresh Fruit and Spinach Salad (page 138).
- At parties, serve fruit wedges with yogurt for dipping.

- Put your microwave to work. Core an apple, pour a couple of tablespoons of orange or lemon juice around it, put a teaspoon of raisins inside, sprinkle with cinnamon, pierce the skin, and cook on high for 5 minutes for a fast baked apple.
- Try grilling fruit. At your next barbecue, put tropical fruit such as pineapple and mango on skewers. Jenny's Caribbean Tuna and Fruit Kebobs (page 198) and the Grilled Banana Splits (page 248) show you how delicious grilled fruit can be.
- Replace some of the fat in baked goods with applesauce. Try the Blueberry Applesauce Muffins (page 68) to taste how delicious low-fat baking can be.
- Keep fruit in a prominent and accessible place—you and your family will eat more than if produce is out of sight.
- Try different varieties of the same fruit—there are so many different kinds of apples and pears, you are bound to find some favorites.
- Be adventuresome and try new fruits—mango, papaya, kiwi, or passionfruit. Many produce sections have free cards with tips on how to use them. Getting kids to try new fruits will help to ensure they will eat them when they are older.

Balsamic Berries

A few drops of aged balsamic vinegar bring out the flavor of the fruit—you won't taste the vinegar.

4 cups strawberries, about 1 pound
1 tablespoon sugar

¼ teaspoon aged balsamic vinegar

1. Wash, dry, hull, and quarter the strawberries lengthwise.

2. Put the strawberries into a large bowl. Add the sugar and balsamic vinegar and toss gently to combine. Refrigerate 1 hour.

3. Spoon the strawberries into chilled stemmed glasses or dessert bowls.

YIELD: 4 servings of 1 cup each

COOK'S NOTE: Aged Italian balsamic vinegar has a more intense flavor than many domestic varieties. Increase the amount to 1 teaspoon if you use the latter.

Nutritional Information Per Serving

Calories 55 | Energy Density 0.37 | Carbohydrate 13 g. | Fat 0 g. | Protein 1 g. | Fiber 3 g.

For a 55-calorie dessert

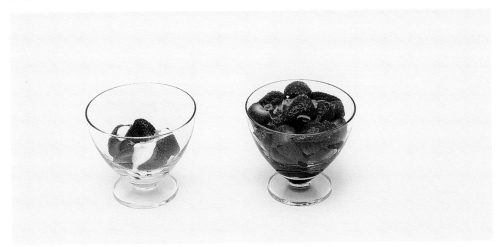

TRADITIONAL	How we lowered the ED	VOLUMETRICS
Strawberries and cream	▸ Substituted balsamic vinegar and a small amount of sugar for cream	Balsamic Berries

Grilled Banana Splits

These make a great ending to a summer evening of grilling.

4 ripe bananas, about ½ pound each
2 tablespoons chocolate chips

½ cup nonfat, frozen vanilla yogurt
4 teaspoons chopped walnuts

1. Preheat a grill or preheat the oven to 400 degrees.

2. Place each banana on its side on a piece of foil. Cut a slit lengthwise across the top. Leave the skin attached.

3. Push ½ tablespoon chocolate chips into the slit of each banana.

4. Wrap the bananas with the foil, leaving the top open. Grill or bake about 15 minutes, or until the chocolate melts.

5. Loosen the foil and press the bananas open a little.

6. Top each banana with 2 tablespoons of the frozen yogurt and sprinkle with 1 teaspoon walnuts.

YIELD: 4 servings

Nutritional Information Per Serving

Calories 185 | Energy Density 1.2 | Carbohydrate 36 g. | Fat 4 g. | Protein 3 g. | Fiber 3 g.

Four-Fruit Compote

Juice and three fruits add up to a refreshing, nonfat dessert. Pictured on page 56.

2 red grapefruit
1 small melon, such as cantaloupe, about
   2¼ pounds
1 cup sliced fresh strawberries

1 tablespoon chopped fresh mint
½ cup orange juice
¾ cup orange sorbet

1. Peel the grapefruit with a knife, making sure to remove all the white pith. Remove the segments between the membranes and place them in a colander to drain.

2. Cut the melon in half and remove the seeds. Scoop out the flesh with a melon baller. There should be about 2 cups melon. Place in a large bowl.

3. Add the strawberries, mint, and grapefruit to the bowl. Pour in the orange juice and stir to combine.

4. Divide the compote among 6 dessert bowls and top each with 2 tablespoons of sorbet.

YIELD: 6 servings of 1½ cups each

COOK'S NOTE: This recipe could also be served, without the sorbet, as part of breakfast, or as a side salad.

Nutritional Information Per Serving

Calories 125 | Energy Density 0.38 | Carbohydrate 28 g. | Fat 0 g. | Protein 2 g. | Fiber 3 g.

Ruby-Red Poached Pears with Raspberry Sauce

Create a light, but grand, finale by poaching one of autumn's most delicious fruits. Pictured on page 4.

6 firm Bartlett pears with stems
1 quart cranberry-apple juice
1 tablespoon lemon juice
3 whole cloves
1 3-inch-long cinnamon stick
1½ cups unsweetened frozen raspberries, thawed

2 tablespoons sugar
½ teaspoon orange liqueur or 1 tablespoon orange juice
6 fresh mint sprigs

1. Carefully peel the pears, leaving the stems intact.

2. Place the juices, cloves, and cinnamon stick in a 4- to 5-quart pot. Lay the pears in the pot and bring to a simmer over medium heat. Simmer the pears, covered, 1 hour.

3. Remove the pot from the heat, uncover, and cool the pears in the liquid. Cover the pot and refrigerate the pears in the liquid overnight.

4. Puree the raspberries, sugar, and liqueur in a food processor or blender. Set the Raspberry Sauce aside.

5. Remove the pears from the liquid. Cut a thin slice from the bottom of each pear.

6. Spoon some of the raspberry sauce on a serving platter or 1 tablespoon on each of 6 dessert plates. Stand the pears on the platter or plates and drizzle 1 tablespoon of the sauce on each pear. Garnish with the mint. Pass any remaining sauce in a small pitcher.

YIELD: 6 servings of 1 pear with about 2 tablespoons of sauce each

COOK'S NOTE: Other cranberry-juice combinations can be substituted for the cranberry-apple. Other frozen berries can be substituted for the raspberries. To produce a clearer sauce and eliminate the seeds, force the raspberry mixture through a fine sieve into a bowl. The sauce provides 8 servings of 2 tablespoons each.

Nutritional Information Per Serving

Calories 125 | Energy Density 0.60 | Carbohydrate 38 g. | Fat 1 g. | Protein 1 g. | Fiber 5 g.

Nutritional Information Per Serving of Sauce

Calories 20 | Energy Density 0.80 | Carbohydrate 5 g. | Fat 0 g. | Protein 0 g. | Fiber 0 g.

Fresh Fruit Parfait

Try this refreshing dessert when fresh berries are in season. It also works well at breakfast. Pictured on the cover.

1½ cups yogurt cheese (page 89)

2 tablespoons honey

½ teaspoon vanilla extract

1 cup sliced fresh strawberries plus
   4 whole, perfect strawberries

1 cup fresh blueberries

1 cup fresh raspberries

4 teaspoons low-fat granola

1. In a mixing bowl, combine the yogurt cheese, honey, and vanilla extract. Beat with an electric mixer until fluffy and smooth.

2. Divide the strawberries among 4 dessert dishes or parfait glasses and top each with 3 tablespoons of the yogurt mixture. Divide the blueberries among the dishes and top each with 3 tablespoons of the yogurt mixture. Divide the raspberries among the dishes and top each with the remaining yogurt mixture. Garnish each parfait with 1 teaspoon of the granola and 1 whole strawberry.

YIELD: 4 servings

Nutritional Information Per Serving

Calories 170 | Energy Density 0.78 | Carbohydrate 32 g. | Fat 0 g. | Protein 11 g. | Fiber 4 g.

For a 170-calorie dessert

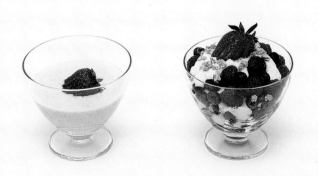

TRADITIONAL	How we lowered the ED	VOLUMETRICS
Strawberry mousse	▸ Used plenty of fresh berries ▸ Substituted yogurt cheese for cream	Fresh Fruit Parfait

Raspberry-Apple Crumble

This updated version of an old favorite uses less butter-filled crumb topping, giving this dessert a lower energy density. Raspberry preserves give it additional flavor.

4 medium, tart apples, such as Granny
   Smith
¼ cup orange juice
2 tablespoons raspberry preserves
2 tablespoons quick-cooking oats
2 tablespoons all-purpose flour

2 tablespoons brown sugar
2 tablespoons wheat germ
½ teaspoon ground cinnamon
Pinch salt
1 tablespoon melted butter

1. Preheat the oven to 350 degrees.

2. Peel, core, and thinly slice the apples.

3. Combine the sliced apples, juice, preserves, and ¼ cup water in a bowl. Pour the mixture into an 8-by-8-inch glass baking dish and set aside.

4. Combine the oats, flour, sugar, wheat germ, cinnamon, and salt. Add the melted butter and mix well.

5. Top the apple mixture with the oats mixture, cover, and bake 1 hour, or until the apples are tender. Uncover the dish for the last 10 minutes of baking.

YIELD: 4 servings of 1 cup each

COOK'S NOTE: Other preserve flavors can be used, such as strawberry or blackberry.

Nutritional Information Per Serving

Calories 175 | Energy Density 1.0 | Carbohydrate 37 g. | Fat 4 g. | Protein 1 g. | Fiber 3 g.

Raspberry-Topped Ricotta Cakes

These delicious individual cheesecakes have only a few ingredients and no measurable fat.

1 cup nonfat ricotta cheese | ⅓ tablespoon honey
2 beaten egg whites | Raspberry Sauce (page 250)

1. Preheat the oven to 350 degrees.

2. Place the ricotta in a bowl and break it up with a wooden spoon. Add the egg whites and honey, and mix until smooth.

3. Lightly coat 4 6-ounce ramekins with cooking spray and divide the ricotta mixture among them. Place the ramekins on a baking sheet and bake for 30 minutes. Cool the ramekins on a wire rack 30 minutes.

4. Run a knife around the edges of the ramekins and unmold onto 4 dessert plates. Spoon 2 tablespoons of Raspberry Sauce around and over each cake.

YIELD: 4 servings

COOK'S NOTE: The cakes can be made ahead and chilled in the refrigerator for an hour or two. Remove from the refrigerator 30 minutes prior to serving.

Nutritional Information Per Serving

Calories 165 | Energy Density 1.1 | Carbohydrate 30 g. | Fat 0 g. | Protein 11 g. | Fiber 1 g.

Strawberry Trifle with Lemon Cream

The classic English dessert has been updated with nonfat yogurt cheese.

3 tablespoons lemon juice
⅔ cup sugar
1 cup Yogurt Cheese (page 89)
4 ounces reduced-fat cream cheese,
   softened
2 teaspoons grated lemon zest

2 teaspoons vanilla extract
2 pints hulled and thinly sliced fresh
   strawberries
12 ladyfingers
Fresh mint sprigs for garnish

1. Combine 2 tablespoons lemon juice and ⅓ cup sugar in a small saucepan and stir over medium heat 3 minutes, or until sugar dissolves. Transfer to a small bowl and set the lemon syrup aside to cool.

2. In a mixing bowl, combine the yogurt cheese, cream cheese, 1 tablespoon lemon juice, lemon zest, vanilla extract, and ⅓ cup sugar. Beat with an electric mixer until fluffy and smooth.

3. Toss the strawberries with 2 tablespoons lemon syrup in a medium bowl.

4. Divide half of the cheese mixture among 6 dessert dishes. Place 1 ladyfinger on each and lightly brush with half the remaining lemon syrup. Top with half the strawberries. Repeat with the remaining cheese mixture, ladyfingers, lemon syrup, and strawberries. Garnish with mint sprigs.

YIELD: 6 servings

COOK'S NOTE: Other berries or combinations of berries can be substituted for the strawberries. You could assemble everything in one serving bowl for a party buffet. Start with half the cheese mixture and 6 ladyfingers and proceed as directed.

Nutritional Information Per Serving

Calories 250 | Energy Density 1.2 | Carbohydrate 43 g. | Fat 5 g. | Protein 8 g. | Fiber 2 g.

For a 250-calorie dessert

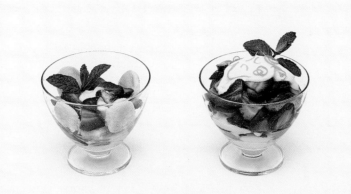

TRADITIONAL	How we lowered the ED	VOLUMETRICS
English trifle with custard sauce	▸ Reduced number of ladyfingers ▸ Used yogurt cheese and reduced-fat cream cheese in place of custard sauce ▸ Added more fruit	Strawberry Trifle with Lemon Cream

Maple Crème Caramel

This is an elegant, easy to make dessert. Be sure to use 100 percent pure maple syrup.

⅓ cup sugar

3 large eggs

1 large egg white

2 cups nonfat milk

½ teaspoon vanilla extract

2 tablespoons 100 percent pure maple syrup

½ teaspoon salt

1. Preheat the oven to 325 degrees.

2. Lightly coat 6 6-ounce ramekins or custard cups with cooking spray.

3. Combine the sugar and 3 tablespoons water in a small, heavy saucepan. Cook, stirring, over medium-high heat until the sugar dissolves. Continue cooking, without stirring, until the mixture turns a deep golden brown, 4 to 8 minutes. Immediately divide the caramel among the ramekins, one at a time, quickly tilting each to coat the bottom and set aside.

4. Whisk the eggs and egg white in a 4-quart measuring cup. Whisk in the milk, vanilla extract, syrup, and salt. Divide the mixture evenly among the ramekins.

5. Place the ramekins in a 13-by-9-inch baking pan and add hot water to a depth of 1 inch. Bake 50 minutes.

6. Cool the ramekins on a rack 30 minutes. Cover the ramekins with plastic wrap and chill, in the refrigerator, 4 hours.

7. Loosen the custards by running a knife around the inside edges of the ramekins. Place a dessert plate upside down over each ramekin and invert the custard onto the plate. Drizzle any remaining caramelized syrup over the custards.

YIELD: 6 servings

Nutritional Information Per Serving

Calories 130 | Energy Density 1.0 | Carbohydrate 19 g. | Fat 3 g. | Protein 6 g. | Fiber 0 g.

Chocolate Fondue with Fresh Fruit

The key to keeping this rich chocolate fondue volumetric is to take a small amount of chocolate with each bite of fruit.

3 ounces semisweet chocolate
2 tablespoons nonfat evaporated milk
1 teaspoon vanilla extract
1 banana, sliced into 1-inch-thick pieces

1 cored and sliced Golden Delicious or
   Granny Smith apple
1 cup halved fresh strawberries
1 cup fresh pineapple chunks

1. Melt the chocolate, milk, and vanilla extract in a fondue pot according to the manufacturer's instructions. If you do not have a fondue pot, melt all the ingredients together in a small saucepan over medium-low heat, stirring constantly. Transfer to a small bowl for serving.

2. Serve the chocolate fondue with the fruit arranged on a plate along with fondue skewers or long toothpicks for dipping.

3. If not serving the fruit immediately, sprinkle a small amount of lemon juice on the apple slices to prevent them from turning brown.

YIELD: 4 servings

COOK'S NOTE: Since the recipe calls for a small amount of chocolate, go ahead and get the best-quality chocolate that you can afford. Try a variety of other fruits such as pears, peaches, orange slices, and raspberries.

Nutritional Information Per Serving

Calories 185 | Energy Density 1.2 | Carbohydrate 33 g. | Fat 6 g. | Protein 3 g. | Fiber 3 g.

Nutritional Information Per Serving of Chocolate Fondue

Calories 114 | Energy Density 3.9 | Carbohydrate 15 g. | Fat 6 g. | Protein 2 g. | Fiber 0 g.

15 Your Personal Eating Plan

In Chapter 2, you estimated your calorie needs and established your daily calorie goals. I am going to give you a menu plan that provides a base of 1400 calories, with suggestions to help you vary the plan to meet *your* specific calorie goal. Remember, you may need to adjust how much you are eating if your weight loss is too fast or too slow. The menu plan is designed to help you achieve your calorie goal by combining foods of different energy densities. You will learn that by including foods low in energy density you can feel satisfied while eating fewer calories than when you first started the plan. After a month of following your menu plan, you will have a good idea of the amounts and types of foods you should be eating. You can then move away from focusing on calories and can concentrate on making nutritious food choices that you enjoy and that help control hunger.

The 1400-calorie plan provides:

- 400-calorie breakfast
- 500-calorie lunch
- 500-calorie dinner

I give you three weeks of menus that provide lots of ideas as to what to eat (pages 269–271). These menus are based on recipes from this book as well as easy-to-prepare meals and convenience foods. The first week of the menu plan heavily emphasizes *Volumetrics* recipes. I know that there will be days when you have little time to cook, so the second week contains a fairly even mix of *Volumetrics* recipes and healthy quick-meal ideas; the third week focuses more on quick-meal ideas and convenience foods. These convenience foods include frozen entrées as well as several meals from fast-food restaurants to give you an idea of the types of foods that are okay occasionally when you are in a hurry. My goal is to show you that you have lots of flexibility to choose menus that fit *your* lifestyle.

You will also notice that I have included a menu for the fourth week, but it is blank (page 272). It will be up to you to develop your own personal *Volumetrics Eating Plan* for this week. You don't have to wait until the end of your third week on the plan to start filling in the foods for Week 4. As you discover volumetric meals and foods that you find particularly appealing, go ahead and add them to your plan for Week 4.

MAKE YOUR OWN PLAN

Don't worry; you don't have to follow the menu plan exactly as it is prescribed. My goal is for you to learn how to incorporate *Volumetrics* eating habits into your lifestyle. I want you to have the skills and confidence to create your own healthful *Volumetrics Eating Plan*. To make it easy for you to follow, I've made the menu plan modular so that you can make substitutions with foods and dishes that have a similar calorie content.

The breakfasts listed in the plan provide 400 calories, while each lunch and dinner provides 500 calories. You will find a list of snack foods to choose from on pages 286–289. For each day, you can pick any breakfast, any lunch, any dinner, and any snacks at your calorie level. You can also interchange a lunch for a dinner or vice versa. I want to give you as much flexibility as possible, so you can make your weight loss plan an enjoyable and sustainable part of your life. For convenience, feel free to use dinner leftovers for lunch the next day. If you like two or three of the lunches, you can stick with these. On the other hand, if you like variety, there are dozens of choices. It's *your* plan.

While I have written this plan to provide 1400 calories a day, it is designed so that you can modify it for whatever calorie level you need. If you decide to go below 1400 calories a day, distribute the reduction across the day. Don't skip meals, and choose foods that provide a balance of nutrients. The table on page 263 provides a strategy to help you use the menu plan to reach your calorie goals.

Achieving your calorie goal

Calorie Level	Strategy
1400 calories	Use the 1400-calorie plan. The menus are for breakfast, lunch, and dinner. If you want to snack, reduce intake at the meals by 100 to 200 calories maximum.
1600 calories	In addition to the foods in the 1400-calorie plan, increase your lunch and dinner from 500 to 600 calories by adding a 100-calorie side dish at each meal, or you can add 200 calories in snacks.
1800 calories	In addition to the foods in the 1400-calorie plan, add 200 calories in snacks. Also, increase your lunch and dinner to 600 calories each by adding a side dish, or increasing the portion size at these meals.
2000 calories	In addition to the foods in the 1400-calorie plan, add 200 calories in snacks. Also, increase your breakfast from 400 to 500 calories and increase your lunch and dinner to 650 calories by adding foods, or increasing the portion size at these meals.
More than 2000 calories	If you need more calories, don't keep adding snacks. Instead, increase portion sizes for breakfast, lunch, and dinner. Main meals contain more protein and more nutrients than most snacks, so this is a healthier approach.

You should use the modular food lists (pages 273–292) to guide your food choices and to eat appropriate amounts. The modular lists include breakfast foods, soups, side dishes, main dishes, desserts, snacks, condiments, and beverages. Within each of these categories, the foods are arranged by calorie level. This makes it easy for you to see foods that have similar calorie levels, so that you can make substitutions. Using these lists, you can modify the menu plan to fit your tastes and food prefer-ences. For example, if you are looking for a 100-calorie side dish, you could pick any side dish that is within the range of 90 to 110 calories. The calories do not have to be exact, so you could choose foods like creamed corn (92 calories) or brown rice (108 calories). You can also substitute other 100-calorie foods or beverages, such as soup or a glass of milk, for the side dish.

Use the modular lists to find ways to vary your calories from the 1400-calorie menu plan. A list of snack foods is provided on pages 286–289 where you can choose 100- or 200-calorie snacks. You can also increase the portions of the foods that you plan to eat for a particular meal. For example, if you need to increase the menu plan by 200 calories, you can double the portion of Tuna and White Bean Salad (page 150). Another option would be to double the portion of the Vegetarian Barley Soup (page 107) to add an extra 120 calories, then choose an additional piece of fruit or a side dish that is around 80 calories.

BEVERAGES

What about beverages? Remember that calories from drinks count. Feel free to have coffee or tea for breakfast, but if you add sugar or cream, you should reduce the calories in the rest of the meal. With the exception of milk, the menus do not include beverages that have calories, such as soft drinks or alcoholic beverages. To save calories, I recommend water or other noncaloric beverages. If you want a soft drink, a glass of juice, a glass of wine, or a beer, have it instead of a snack (12 ounces of soda or juice contain about 150 calories).

Milk is an excellent source of protein and calcium. Our breakfasts, with low-fat milk or yogurt, are rich in calcium, and lunches and dinners include dairy foods, but drinking low-fat or nonfat milk is a good idea as well. An 8-ounce glass of nonfat milk has about 85 calories; the same amount of 1 percent milk has around 100 calories. If you are on the 2000-calorie plan, you can have a glass of milk with the basic 500-calorie lunch or dinner to reach your desired 600 calories. Or have a glass of milk with a 100-calorie snack to count for a 200-calorie snack.

CALCIUM AND SALT

By now you know a lot about how to eat volumetrically. You are eating more low-energy-dense foods such as fruits, vegetables, and soups, and making sure you get adequate amounts of satiety enhancing lean protein and fiber. You also need to get enough calcium. If you realize you are not able to fit three calcium-rich foods, such as milk, yogurt, and cheese, into your menu plan, you should consider taking a calcium supplement.

While you are looking for more calcium, you should also check out the sodium content of foods on the nutrition facts label. Health organizations such as the American Diabetes Association and the American Heart Association recommend no more than 2400 mg of sodium per day. I have not discussed salt in foods because it does not affect body fat. If you are concerned about your salt intake or if you have been told to restrict it because you have high blood pressure, then you should limit added salt and eat fewer processed foods or find reduced-salt versions. For example, use reduced-salt soup, or if you are using canned beans, rinse them thoroughly.

VARIETY AND AFFORDABILITY

As you look through the recipes, you will notice there is lots of variety. I have included many dishes that can be prepared quickly, such as Stir-fried Beef with Snow Peas and Cherry Tomatoes (page 181), Chicken Parmesan (page 205), Shrimp Creole (page 199), and Balsamic Berries (page 246). You will also find some dishes that need a little more time in the kitchen and are perfect for special occasions. Some of the dishes fit well into a tight budget, such as Curried Cauliflower Soup (page 100), Tuna and White Bean Salad (page 150), Bayou Red Beans and Rice (page 218), and Spaghetti with Tomato and Fresh Basil Sauce (page 233). Again, this is *your* plan; feel free to modify the recipes to fit your taste, schedule, and budget.

The Volumetrics Eating Plan is meant to be adapted to fit into any lifestyle. The Lehman family tells you about how they have incorporated *Volumetrics* into their daily routine:

> *As a young couple with a busy lifestyle, we needed an eating plan that was both balanced and easy to follow. We stumbled upon a magazine article featuring the Volumetrics concepts and decided to read The Volumetrics Weight-Control Plan. Volumetrics made sense to us from a scientific perspective and offered a great deal of flexibility and variety—exactly what we were looking for. It's been over a year now and we still subscribe to the plan. It's simply become part of our lifestyle . . . and best of all, we feel great and are never hungry between meals!*
>
> *Dan and Ann Lehman*

Following the *Volumetrics Eating Plan* doesn't have to be expensive. Use these tips to save money at the grocery store.

- Make substitutions in recipes. For example, use:
  - frozen fish instead of fresh fish
  - canola oil instead of olive oil
  - frozen or canned vegetables instead of fresh
- Use leftovers in soups and casseroles.
- Take advantage of fresh produce when it is in season. Plant your own vegetable garden outdoors or plant an herb container-garden indoors.
- Shop when you have time to read labels and compare prices. Choose store brands instead of national brands.
- Make use of the sales circulars and coupons. Plan your meals from items you bought on sale or with a coupon. Stock up on staples when they are on sale. This may take a bit of time and organization, but can help your grocery dollars go farther.
- Buy in bulk. Many times items sold in large quantities are offered at discounted prices. Careful, though, check out the price per unit! Just because it is a big box doesn't necessarily mean it's cheaper.
- Eat before you shop, and take a list of what you need so you won't be tempted to make impulse purchases.

A LIFETIME OF HEALTHY EATING

Once you have achieved your weight loss, you can use this plan for maintenance, which, for some, may be more of a challenge than losing weight. After following the plan for a month, you should have learned how much you can eat to keep calories at the right level. By that time, I hope this way of eating won't feel like a program for you. It will be the way you enjoy eating. A few more tips:

- At any meal, you can eat more vegetables (except starchy ones like potatoes and corn, or vegetables that are covered in butter, oil, or high-fat sauce) while only slightly increasing your calorie intake.
- Don't worry about counting portions or calories exactly, especially of foods that have a very low- or low-energy density. The plan is designed to maintain the appropriate calorie levels, but you don't have to measure everything perfectly for this weight-loss plan to work.
- Because these meals aren't full of special diet foods, it's easy to share them with a spouse, a friend, or family members. If they aren't restricting calories to lose weight, they can increase their portions.

My goal is to show you a nutritious way of eating that can fill you up on fewer calories, so you can lose weight without a feeling of deprivation. Even more important, I want to show you how enjoyable healthy eating can be. To remind you of what you have learned about eating the *Volumetrics* way, I have put together a summary of the basics on page 268.

Summary of the *Volumetrics Eating Plan*

Foods	Recommendations
Water-rich Foods	Consume more foods with a high-water content. You can usually eat satisfying portions of these foods, which will help you to feel full with very few calories. Foods high in water content include: • Fruits and vegetables, with little or no added sugar or fat • Soups and stews • Casseroles with plenty of vegetables • Hot cereals and cooked grains • Steamed or poached fish Eat more vegetables and fruits at meals and for snacks. Start a meal with fresh fruit, soup or salad.
Low-fat Foods	Fat is high in energy density, so finding ways to reduce the fat in your diet and in your recipes will help to lower the energy density. Here are a few suggestions: • Reduce the amount of high-fat spreads, dressings, and sauces that you eat. • Substitute commonly used high-fat items with low-fat items. • Choose low-fat dairy products. • Choose low-fat fish, poultry, meat, egg whites, or beans. • Minimize how often you eat fried foods. Bake, steam, grill, or broil instead. • Substitute low-fat desserts, snacks, and beverages for high-fat items.
Portions	To decrease calorie intake and feel full on fewer calories, choose satisfying portions of very low- and low-energy-dense foods. Have smaller portions of medium- and high-energy-dense foods, when you choose them.
Fiber-rich Foods	Fiber moderately lowers energy density, but most importantly it increases your feeling of fullness. The following types of foods will fit into your low-energy-dense diet: • Whole fruits and vegetables with little or no added fat or sugar. • Whole grains, like whole-wheat bread or brown rice. • Fiber-rich breakfast cereals (hot or cold) with little or no added sugar.
Lean Protein Foods	Lean protein is very satisfying and will also help you to feel full. Make low-energy-dense choices such as: • Low-fat fish • Poultry without skin • Lean meats • Beans and tofu Combine protein with low-energy-dense vegetables, grains, and fruits.
Low-calorie Beverages	Choose your beverages wisely. Watch your intake of sugary drinks and alcohol, which add calories with little fullness. Replace sugary drinks with water, black coffee, or other low-calorie beverages.

WEEK 1 Menu Plan: The meals listed in this first week contain a variety of *Volumetrics* recipes. Feel free to try meals from weeks 2 and 3 or to make substitutions with the modular lists.

Monday	Tuesday	Wednesday	Thursday	Friday	Saturday	Sunday
Breakfast	**Breakfast**	**Breakfast**	**Breakfast**	**Breakfast**	**Breakfast**	**Breakfast**
1 cup wheat bran flakes ½ cup blueberries 1 banana (302 calories) 1 cup 1% milk (102 calories)	1 whole-wheat English muffin 1 ounce Swiss cheese (220 calories) 1 grapefruit ½ teaspoon sugar (81 calories) 1 cup 1% milk (102 calories)	1 packet instant oatmeal ¼ cup oat bran ¼ cup raisins dash cinnamon (307 calories) 1 cup 1% milk (102 calories)	2 whole-wheat frozen waffles 1 tablespoon light margarine ½ cup strawberries 1 kiwifruit (292 calories) 1 cup 1% milk (102 calories)	1½ cups oat bran flakes ¼ cup dried cranberries (296 calories) 1 cup 1% milk (102 calories)	*Creamy Apricot Oatmeal* (page 69, 265 calories) ½ pink grapefruit ¼ teaspoon sugar (40 calories) 1 cup 1% milk (102 calories)	*Piquant Frittata* (page 66, 175 calories) 1 cup cantaloupe 1 cup honeydew (118 calories) 1 cup 1% milk (102 calories)
Lunch	**Lunch**	**Lunch**	**Lunch**	**Lunch**	**Lunch**	**Lunch**
Roasted Portobello Sandwich (page 119, 290 calories) *Tabbouleh* (page 148, 100 calories) 1 pear (98 calories)	*Cold-Cut Combo Sandwich* (page 116, 345 calories) *Tangy Cole Slaw* (page 139, 65 calories) ½ cup fruit-flavored gelatin 1 cup strawberries (80 calories)	*Garden Fresh Vegetable Pizza* (page 238, 285 calories) *Gazpacho* (page 110, 120 calories) 1 snack cup nonfat chocolate pudding (100 calories)	*Zesty Tuna Salad Pita* (page 124, 285 calories) *Fresh Fruit and Spinach Salad with Orange-Poppy Seed Dressing* (page 138, 150 calories) 1 apple (81 calories)	*South of the Border Chicken Stew* (page 208, 325 calories) *Volumetrics Salad* (page 134, 100 calories) 1 cup fruit cocktail in light syrup (76 calories)	*Santa Fe Steak Salad* (page 144, 400 calories) ½ cup low-fat cottage cheese ¼ cup peaches canned in light syrup (108 calories)	*Risotto Primavera* (page 222, 290 calories) *Fennel, Orange, & Arugula Salad* (page 133, 80 calories) *Maple Créme Caramel* (page 258, 130 calories)
Dinner	**Dinner**	**Dinner**	**Dinner**	**Dinner**	**Dinner**	**Dinner**
Chicken Merlot (page 206, 240 calories) ⅔ cup brown rice (144 calories) *Insalata Mista* (page 137, 60 calories) *Balsamic Berries* (page 246, 55 calories)	*Veggie-Stuffed Macaroni and Cheese* (page 234, 330 calories) *Curried Cauliflower Soup* (page 100, 105 calories) ¾ cup mandarin orange slices (69 calories)	*Baked Tilapia with Sautéed Vegetables* (page 194, 160 calories) *Oven Roasted Potatoes* (page 169, 110 calories) *Roasted Asparagus* (page 163, 50 calories) *Chocolate Fondue with Fresh Fruit* (page 259, 185 calories)	*South of the Border Chicken Stew* (page 208, 325 calories) Whole-wheat roll (110 calories) 1 cup grapes (62 calories)	*Poach-Roast Salmon* (page 193, 225 calories) *Vegetable Pilaf* (page 221, 135 calories) *Charlie's Greek Salad* (page 130, 80 calories) 1 3-ounce frozen fruit and juice bar (70 calories)	*Charlie's Pasta Primavera* (page 228, 345 calories) *Corn & Tomato Chowder* (page 95, 105 calories) 1 kiwifruit (46 calories)	*Pork Chops with Orange-Soy Sauce* (page 188, 195 calories) *Stir-Fried Green Beans* (page 164, 65 calories) ½ cup brown rice (72 calories) *Raspberry-Topped Ricotta Cakes* (page 255, 165 calories)

WEEK 2 Menu Plan: Here you will find a mix of Volumetrics recipes and quick meal ideas.

Monday	Tuesday	Wednesday	Thursday	Friday	Saturday	Sunday
Breakfast	**Breakfast**	**Breakfast**	**Breakfast**	**Breakfast**	**Breakfast**	**Breakfast**
1 packet instant maple & brown sugar oatmeal ¼ cup oat bran (235 calories) 1 orange (62 calories) 1 cup 1% milk (102 calories)	1½ cups wheat bran flake cereal 1 peach (246 calories) 1 cup cantaloupe (56 calories) 1 cup 1% milk (102 calories)	1 cup nonfat vanilla yogurt 1 cup pineapple ¼ cup low-fat granola (304 calories) 1 cup 1% milk (102 calories)	2 cups shredded wheat cereal ¼ cup dried apricots (291 calories) 1 cup 1% milk (102 calories)	1 whole-wheat English muffin 1 tablespoon reduced-fat peanut butter 1 sliced apple (304 calories) 1 cup 1% milk (102 calories)	*Jennifer's Fruit-Smothered Whole-Wheat Buttermilk Pancakes* (page 62, 270 calories) 1 cup sugar-free fruited yogurt (120 calories)	*Mexican Egg Wrap* (page 65, 240 calories) 1 cup grapes (62 calories) 1 cup 1% milk (102 calories)
Lunch	**Lunch**	**Lunch**	**Lunch**	**Lunch**	**Lunch**	**Lunch**
1 baked potato topped with veggies, salsa, and cheese (350 calories) *Lemony Fennel Salad* (page 136, 55 calories) 1 pear (98 calories)	6" turkey sub on a wheat roll (no mayo or cheese, but lots of veggies) (280 calories) 2 cups vegetarian vegetable soup (144 calories) 1 cup grapes (81 calories)	*Buffalo Chicken Wrap* (page 120, 350 calories) *Insalata Mista* (page 137, 60 calories) 1 apple (81 calories)	*Tuna and White Bean Salad* (page 150, 200 calories) 1 3½-inch oat bran bagel (181 calories) 1 cup sugar-free fruited yogurt (120 calories)	1 frozen reduced-calorie entrée of choice (300 calories) 15 baby carrots 1 tablespoon nonfat ranch dressing (82 calories) 1 banana (109 calories)	*Open-Faced Roast Beef Sandwich* (page 118, 200 calories) *Cannellini Bean Soup* (page 105, 265 calories) 1 plum (40 calories)	*Ratatouille* (page 162, 75 calories) 1 cup whole-wheat pasta (174 calories) *Strawberry Trifle with Lemon Cream* (page 256, 250 calories)
Dinner	**Dinner**	**Dinner**	**Dinner**	**Dinner**	**Dinner**	**Dinner**
Old World Goulash (page 182, 335 calories) *Stuffed Mushrooms Florentine* (page 86, 45 calories) ½ cup low-fat cottage cheese 1 kiwifruit (128 calories)	*Bayou Red Beans & Rice* (page 218, 300 calories) *Volumetrics Salad* (page 134, 100 calories) ½ cup low-fat vanilla ice cream (92 calories)	¾ cup cooked whole-wheat pasta, 1⅓ cups frozen mixed vegetables, ½ cup prepared pasta sauce, and 1 teaspoon Parmesan cheese (460 calories) Piece of chocolate (50 calories)	*Hearty Chicken and Vegetable Soup* (page 108, 290 calories) *Fresh Fruit and Spinach Salad with Orange-Poppy Seed Dressing* (page 138, 150 calories) 1 cup cantaloupe (56 calories)	*Nouveau Lamb Stew* (page 186, 245 calories) *Insalata Caprese* (page 81, 105 calories) ½ cup chocolate pudding (150 calories)	*Oceanside Pasta* (page 230, 400 calories) *Creamy Cucumber and Dill Salad* (page 132, 50 calories) ½ cup peaches ½ tablespoon reduced-fat frozen whipped topping (51 calories)	*Stir-Fried Beef with Snow Peas and Cherry Tomatoes* (page 181, 255 calories) *Asian Spring Rolls* (page 82, 130 calories) 2 fortune cookies (56 calories) ½ peach 1 tablespoon light cream (51 calories)

WEEK 3 Menu Plan: This week contains a variety of quick meal ideas along with several Volumetrics recipes.

Monday	Tuesday	Wednesday	Thursday	Friday	Saturday	Sunday
Breakfast	**Breakfast**	**Breakfast**	**Breakfast**	**Breakfast**	**Breakfast**	**Breakfast**
2 slices whole-wheat toast 2 tablespoons reduced-fat cream cheese 2 kiwifruits (292 calories) 1 cup 1% milk (102 calories)	2 eggs scrambled 2 tablespoons salsa (163 calories) ¾ cup pineapple ½ cup low-fat cottage cheese (139 calories) 1 cup 1% milk (102 calories)	1 cup nonfat vanilla yogurt ¾ cup chopped mango ¼ cup low-fat granola (309 calories) 1 cup 1% milk (102 calories)	2 cups shredded wheat cereal 1 diced peach (256 calories) 1 tangerine (37 calories) 1 cup 1% milk (102 calories)	2 veggie sausage links (80 calories) 2 slices whole-wheat toast, ½ tablespoon light margarine (155 calories) 1 cup honeydew (62 calories) 1 cup 1% milk (102 calories)	2 Blueberry Applesauce Muffins (page 68, 250 calories) ½ pink grapefruit ¼ teaspoon sugar (40 calories) 1 cup 1% milk (102 calories)	Baked Berry French Toast (page 64, 315 calories) ¾ cup 1% milk (75 calories)
Lunch	**Lunch**	**Lunch**	**Lunch**	**Lunch**	**Lunch**	**Lunch**
Grilled chicken sandwich (no mayo or cheese, but lots of veggies) (320 calories) 7 wheat crackers, 1 ounce reduced-fat cheese (144 calories) 1 clementine (37 calories)	5-ounce frozen bean and cheese burrito ¼ cup salsa (325 calories) 1 cup sugar-free fruited yogurt 1 cup strawberries (168 calories)	Ham sandwich on 6" wheat roll, 1 slice cheese (no mayo, but lots of veggies) (380 calories) ½ cup fruit sorbet (120 calories)	1 can broth-based vegetable soup (180 calories) 1 whole-wheat bagel 1 tablespoon reduced-fat cream cheese (230 calories) 1 pear (98 calories)	1 frozen reduced-calorie entrée of choice (300 calories) 1½ cups chicken, rice, and vegetable soup (135 calories) 1 cup grapes (62 calories)	1 small fast-food cheeseburger (no mayo, but lots of veggies) (310 calories) Large garden salad without croutons, ¼ cup fat-free salad dressing (150 calories) 1 plum (40 calories)	Veggie burger on a whole-wheat roll, lettuce and sliced tomato (320 calories) 2 cups chicken noodle soup (150 calories) ½ cup raspberries (30 calories)
Dinner	**Dinner**	**Dinner**	**Dinner**	**Dinner**	**Dinner**	**Dinner**
¼ of a bagged, reduced-calorie, frozen family-size meal entrée. Add 2 cups frozen vegetables (300 calories) 1 ounce angel food cake, ½ cup strawberries, 2 tablespoons reduced-calorie whipped topping (193 calories)	Chicken Fajita Pizza (page 240, 390 calories) ½ cup sugar-free vanilla pudding prepared with nonfat milk ½ cup blueberries (110 calories)	Pizza Margherita (page 239, 265 calories) Green salad with nonfat dressing (50 calories) Grilled Banana Splits (page 248, 185 calories)	Shrimp Fried Rice (page 200, 325 calories) 1 cup fresh pineapple (76 calories) 1 fortune cookie (28 calories) ½ cup nonfat frozen yogurt (80 calories)	Liz's Pasta Salad (page 146, 400 calories) Baked apple, 1 teaspoon sugar, dash of cinnamon (96 calories)	3-ounce baked pork chop 1 cup wild rice (338 calories) White Bean Bruschetta (page 79, 60 calories) Minted broccoli (page 158, 35 calories) 1¼ cups watermelon (60 calories)	Italian Turkey Spirals (page 212, 140 calories) 1 cup green beans (20 calories) ¾ cup brown rice (162 calories) Fresh Fruit Parfait (page 252, 170 calories)

WEEK 4 Menu Plan: Fill this in with your favorite Volumetrics meals

Monday	Tuesday	Wednesday	Thursday	Friday	Saturday	Sunday
Breakfast	**Breakfast**	**Breakfast**	**Breakfast**	**Breakfast**	**Breakfast**	**Breakfast**
Lunch	Lunch	Lunch	Lunch	Lunch	Lunch	Lunch
Dinner	Dinner	Dinner	Dinner	Dinner	Dinner	Dinner

MODULAR FOOD LISTS

You can use these lists to make substitutions for foods in the menu plan and when developing your personal Volumetrics Eating Plan. Within each modular list, foods are grouped by calorie level, so you can easily determine which foods are interchangeable. The energy density of each food is listed to help you make the most satiating choices. I've also included the weight of the foods in grams so you will see how the portion sizes compare when you are choosing foods. To find the values for more foods, check *The Volumetrics Weight-Control Plan*.

Breakfast Food Modular List

Let's use the breakfast modular list to show you how to make the most satiating choices. When choosing between foods with a similar calorie level, you will be able to have a larger portion if you choose the food with the lower energy density. For example, a glazed doughnut (E.D. 4.0) and the Creamy Apricot Oatmeal (page 69) (E.D. 0.90) both contain about 250 calories. The doughnut weighs 61 grams; the oatmeal weighs 294 grams—almost 5 times as much.

Cereal with nonfat or low-fat milk is a good choice for breakfast. Check the label to find cereals you like that have at least 3 grams of fiber per serving. Pay attention to portion sizes. I list calories per cup of cereal, but that does not mean you should eat that amount. If you ate a cup of granola with milk, you would consume 620 calories!

	Energy Density	Weight (grams)	Calories
Less than 100 calories			
Scrambled liquid egg substitute, ¼ cup	0.91	58	53
Whole-wheat toast, 1 slice	2.8	23	65
White toast, 1 slice	2.9	23	67
Poached egg, 1 large egg	1.5	50	75
Boiled egg, 1 large egg	1.6	49	78
Turkey kielbasa, 2 ounces	1.4	57	80
Veggie sausage links, 2 links	1.8	45	80
Pancake, 1 plain item, 4-inch diameter	2.3	37	86
Waffle, 1 plain, frozen variety	2.6	33	87
Canadian bacon, 2 slices	1.9	47	89
Turkey bacon, 3 slices	2.4	37	90
Fried egg, 1 large egg	2.0	46	92
100 to 200 calories			
Cream of Wheat, 1 cup, prepared with water	0.49	251	123
Blueberry Applesauce Muffins, page 68	1.6	78	125
English muffin, toasted	2.6	51	128
Pork bacon, 3 slices	5.7	24	138
Corn grits, 1 cup, prepared with water	0.60	242	145
Oatmeal, 1 cup, instant, prepared with water	0.62	233	145
Kellogg's Product 19 cereal, 1 cup with ½ cup 1 percent milk	1.0	151	151
Corn flakes cereal, 1 cup with ½ cup 1 percent milk	1.1	137	151
French toast, 1 slice, made with 2 percent milk	2.3	66	151
Bran muffin, 2½-inch diameter	2.7	57	153
Shredded wheat cereal, small biscuit, 1 cup with ½ cup 1 percent milk	1.4	113	158
General Mills Wheaties, 1 cup with ½ cup 1 percent milk	1.1	146	161
General Mills Cheerios, 1 cup with ½ cup of 1 percent milk	1.1	147	162
General Mills Fiber One cereal, 1 cup with ½ cup 1 percent milk	0.94	182	171
Piquant Frittata, page 66	1.0	170	175
Oat bran bagel, 1 item, 3⅓-inch diameter	2.5	70	181
Post Grape-Nuts Flakes cereal, 1 cup with ½ cup 1 percent milk	1.1	168	185

	Energy Density	Weight (grams)	Calories
Cinnamon raisin bagel, 3⅓-inch diameter	2.9	67	194
Plain bagel, 3⅓-inch diameter	2.8	70	195
Oat bran flakes cereal, 1 cup with ½ cup 1 percent milk	1.2	165	198

200 to 300 calories

	Energy Density	Weight (grams)	Calories
Wheat bran flakes cereal, 1 cup with ½ cup 1 percent milk	1.2	170	204
Fruit toaster pastry	3.9	52	204
All-bran cereal, Kellogg's, 1 cup with ½ cup 1 percent milk	1.1	192	211
1 biscuit, 2½-inch diameter	3.5	61	212
Cinnamon sweet roll with raisins	3.7	60	223
Post 100 percent Bran cereal, 1 cup with ½ cup 1 percent milk	1.2	188	226
Butter croissant	4.1	56	231
Mexican Egg Wrap, page 65	1.3	185	240
Quaker Toasted oatmeal cereal, 1 cup with ½ cup 1 percent milk	1.4	171	240
Raisin bran cereal, 1 cup with ½ cup 1 percent milk	1.3	185	241
Glazed doughnut	4.0	61	242
General Mills Multibran Chex cereal, 1 cup with ½ cup 1 percent milk	1.4	179	251
Creamy Apricot Oatmeal, page 69	0.90	294	265
Jennifer's Fruit-Smothered Whole-Wheat Buttermilk Pancakes, page 62	1.0	230	270

300 to 400 calories

	Energy Density	Weight (grams)	Calories
Baked Berry French Toast, page 64	1.1	286	315
Cinnamon Danish pastry, 1 item	4.0	87	349
Butter croissant with bacon, eggs, and cheese	3.3	117	386

More than 400 calories

	Energy Density	Weight (grams)	Calories
Granola cereal, 1 cup, reduced-fat, with ½ cup 1 percent milk	2.0	216	431
Post Grape-nuts cereal, 1 cup with ½ cup 1 percent milk	1.9	237	451
Pork sausage, 2 fried patties	6.7	76	506
Biscuit with egg and sausage	3.2	182	581
Granola cereal, 1 cup with ½ cup 1 percent milk	2.5	248	620

Soup Modular List

Remember, if you are choosing a soup as a starter, keep the calories to 150 or less. Soups that are higher in calories make a nutritious and filling main course at lunch or dinner. Soups also make good snacks. If you are buying prepared soup, check the label for the energy density and calories since brands can differ considerably.

	Energy Density	Weight (grams)	Calories
Less than 100 calories			
Chicken broth, 1 cup, nonfat	0.07	243	17
Beef broth, 1 cup, nonfat	0.08	250	20
Vegetable broth, 1 cup	0.09	222	20
Beef broth, 1 cup	0.12	250	30
Chicken broth, 1 cup	0.16	244	39
Gazpacho, 1 cup, canned, ready to serve	0.23	243	56
Onion soup, 1 cup, canned, condensed, prepared with water	0.24	242	58
Vegetarian vegetable soup, 1 cup, canned, condensed, prepared with water	0.30	240	72
Chicken noodle soup, 1 cup, canned, condensed, prepared with water	0.31	242	75
Minestrone soup, 1 cup, canned, condensed, prepared with water	0.34	241	82
Tomato soup, 1 cup, canned, condensed, prepared with water	0.35	243	85
Chicken, rice and vegetable soup, 1 cup canned, ready to serve	0.38	237	90
New England clam chowder, 1 cup canned, condensed, prepared with water	0.39	244	95
100 to 200 calories			
Curried Cauliflower Soup, page 100	0.30	350	105
Corn and Tomato Chowder, page 95	0.40	263	105
Black bean soup, 1 cup, canned, condensed, prepared with water	0.47	247	116
Gazpacho, page 110	0.28	429	120
Vegetarian Barley Soup, page 107	0.40	300	120

	Energy Density	Weight (grams)	Calories
Vegetable soup, 1 cup, canned, ready-to-serve	0.51	239	122
Rustic Tomato Soup, page 101	0.40	312	125
Minestrone, page 102	0.50	250	125
Lentil and ham soup, 1 cup, canned, ready-to-serve	0.56	248	139
Autumn Harvest Pumpkin Soup, page 96	0.40	375	150
Beef with vegetables, 1 cup, canned, ready-to-serve	0.63	243	153
Creamy Broccoli Soup, page 98	0.60	267	160
Tomato soup, 1 cup canned condensed, prepared with 2 percent milk	0.65	248	161
Beef soup, 1 cup, canned, ready-to-serve	0.71	239	170
Bean with bacon soup, 1 cup, canned, condensed, prepared with water	0.68	253	172
Chicken noodle, 1 cup, canned, ready-to-serve	0.73	240	175
Split pea soup with ham, 1 cup	0.77	240	185
Potato ham chowder, 1 cup, canned, ready-to-serve	0.80	240	192
Corn chowder, 1 cup, canned, ready-to-serve	0.82	244	200

More than 200 calories

	Energy Density	Weight (grams)	Calories
Cream of mushroom soup, 1 cup, canned, condensed, prepared with 2 percent milk	0.82	248	203
Lentil and Tomato Soup, page 106	0.60	383	230
Bean with ham soup, 1 cup canned, ready-to-serve	0.95	243	231
Asian Black Bean Soup, page 104	0.70	343	240
Cannellini Bean Soup, page 105	0.50	470	265
Hearty Chicken and Vegetable Soup, page 108	0.60	483	290

Side Dish Modular List

This list contains an assortment of side dishes such as vegetables, grains, salads, and starters. You will find many dishes of less than 100 calories, as well as many in the 100 to 200 calorie range. I've included a few side dishes with calorie levels greater than 200 calories; they can also be used as main dishes.

	Energy Density	Weight (grams)	Calories
Less than 100 calories			
Cauliflower, ½ cup, boiled	0.23	61	14
Green cabbage, ½ cup, boiled	0.23	74	17
Summer squash, ½ cup, boiled	0.20	90	18
Swiss chard, ½ cup, boiled	0.20	90	18
Spinach, ½ cup, boiled	0.22	95	21
Green beans, ½ cup, boiled	0.35	62	22
Asparagus, ½ cup, boiled	0.24	92	22
Carrots, ½ cup, raw	0.43	61	26
Brussels sprouts, ½ cup, boiled	0.39	77	30
Minted Broccoli, page 158	0.28	125	35
Beets, ½ cup, boiled	0.44	84	37
Winter squash, ½ cup, baked	0.39	102	40
Stuffed Mushrooms Florentine, page 86	0.40	113	45
Creamy Cucumber and Dill Salad, page 132	0.28	179	50
Roasted Asparagus, page 163	0.40	125	50
Lemony Fennel Salad, page 136	0.36	153	55
Insalata Mista, page 137	0.39	154	60
White Bean Bruschetta, page 79	1.5	50	60
Green peas, ½ cup, frozen, boiled	0.78	79	62
Stir-Fried Green Beans, page 164	0.40	163	65
Pepper Slaw, page 140	0.60	108	65
Tangy Coleslaw, page 139	0.43	151	65
Corn, ½ cup, canned, boiled	0.81	81	66
Ratatouille, page 162	0.50	150	75
Bulgur, ½ cup, cooked	0.83	92	76

	Energy Density	Weight (grams)	Calories
Cob of corn, 1 item, boiled	0.86	90	77
Buckwheat grouts (kasha), ½ cup, roasted, cooked	0.97	79	77
Charlie's Greek Salad, page 130	0.50	160	80
Fennel, Orange, and Arugula Salad, page 133	0.58	138	80
Cowpeas (black-eyed peas), ½ cup, boiled	0.97	82	80
Garlic-Roasted Vegetables, page 160	0.40	225	90
Sesame Mushroom Kebobs, page 84	0.70	129	90
French fried potatoes, 1 ounce	3.2	28	91
Refried beans, ½ cup, canned, nonfat	0.72	128	92
Creamed corn, ½ cup	0.72	128	92
Lima beans, ½ cup, frozen, boiled	1.1	86	95
Pearled barley, ½ cup, cooked	1.2	81	97

100 to 200 calories

	Energy Density	Weight (grams)	Calories
Volumetrics Salad, page 134	0.30	333	100
Black beans, ½ cup, canned	0.78	128	100
Tabbouleh, page 148	1.0	100	100
Kidney beans, ½ cup, canned	0.81	128	104
Insalata Caprese, page 81	0.81	130	105
Quinoa, ½ cup, cooked	0.99	107	106
Lima beans, ½ cup, boiled	1.2	90	108
Brown rice, ½ cup, cooked	1.1	98	108
Oven-Roasted Potatoes, page 169	1.6	69	110
Mashed potatoes with margarine and whole milk, ½ cup	1.1	101	111
Lentils, ½ cup, boiled	1.2	96	115
Split peas, ½ cup, boiled	1.2	96	115
Sweet potato, ½ cup, baked	1.0	117	117
Pinto beans, ½ cup, boiled	1.4	84	117
Refried beans, ½ cup, canned	0.94	127	119
Navy beans, ½ cup, boiled	1.4	92	129
Asian Spring Rolls, page 82	1.2	108	130
New Potatoes with Peas, page 168	0.80	169	135
Vegetable Pilaf, page 221	0.90	150	135
Chickpeas (garbanzo beans), ½ cup, canned	1.2	119	143
Millet, ½ cup, cooked	1.2	119	143
Bulgur-and-Vegetable-Stuffed Peppers, page 172	0.50	300	150

	Energy Density	Weight (grams)	Calories
Fresh Fruit and Spinach Salad, page 138	0.64	234	150
Great Northern beans, ½ cup, canned	1.1	136	150
White beans, ½ cup, canned	1.2	128	154
Potato Salad with Green Beans and Tarragon, page 149	0.80	194	155
Smashed Potatoes, page 170	0.90	211	155
Hash-brown potatoes, ½ cup	2.1	78	163
Baked beans, ½ cup, homemade	1.5	127	191
Mary's Quinoa with Lime, page 224	0.77	253	195
More than 200 calories			
Herbed Barley Stuffed Squash, page 171	0.60	350	210
Baked potato with skin, 1 medium	1.1	193	212
Lemon Shrimp Bruschetta, page 80	1.6	134	215
Onion rings, 7 batter-dipped rings, fried	4.1	70	285

Main Dish Modular List

In this list you will find a variety of dishes that serve as the center of the meal. They are varied and include meat, poultry and fish, as well as pizza, pasta, sandwiches, and large salads. Add side dishes and starters that fit your calorie level and balance your meal.

	Energy Density	Weight (grams)	Calories
Less than 100 calories			
Orange roughy, 3 ounces, cooked with dry heat	0.89	85	76
Alaskan king crab, 3 ounces, cooked with moist heat	0.96	85	82
Lobster, 3 ounces, cooked with moist heat	0.98	85	83
Shrimp, 3 ounces, boiled or steamed	1.0	84	84
Cod, 3 ounces, cooked with dry heat	1.0	89	89
Scallops, 3 ounces, cooked with moist heat	1.1	82	90
Tuna, 3 ounces, canned in water	1.2	83	99
100 to 200 calories			
Perch, 3 ounces, cooked with dry heat	1.2	83	100
Turkey tenderloin, 3 ounces	1.3	85	110
Oysters, 3 ounces, cooked with moist heat	1.4	83	116
Yellowfin tuna, 3 ounces, cooked with dry heat	1.4	84	118
Halibut, 3 ounces, cooked with dry heat	1.4	85	119
Turkey breast, ground, 4 ounces, 99 percent fat-free	1.4	86	120
Clams, 3 ounces, cooked with moist heat	1.5	84	126
Pink salmon, 3 ounces, cooked with dry heat	1.5	85	127
Swordfish, 3 ounces, broiled with margarine	1.6	83	132
Chicken liver, 3.5 ounces, simmered	1.6	83	133
Italian Turkey Spirals, page 212	1.0	140	140
Roasted Lamb Chops with Gremolata, page 190	1.3	108	140
Cheese pizza, 1 slice, ⅛ of 12-inch-diameter pie, regular crust	2.2	64	140
Chicken breast, 3.5 ounces, roasted, no skin	1.7	84	142
Ham, 3.5 ounces, extra lean (5 percent fat)	1.5	97	145
Cornish game hen, ½ bird, without skin	1.4	105	147
Vegetable pizza, 1 slice, ⅛ of 12-inch-diameter pie, thin crust	2.1	70	148
Turkey, 3.5 ounces, white meat without skin	1.6	98	157
Baked Tilapia with Sautéed Vegetables, page 194	0.80	200	160
Turkey, 3.5 ounces, ground, lean 7 percent fat	1.9	84	160
Beef liver, 3.5 ounces, braised	1.6	101	161
Chicken Provençal, page 210	0.70	236	165
Tuna, 3 ounces, canned in oil	2.0	84	168
Oysters, 3 ounces, breaded and fried	2.0	84	168
Clams, 3 ounces, breaded and fried	2.0	86	172
Macaroni, 1 cup, whole-wheat, cooked	1.2	145	174

	Energy Density	Weight (grams)	Calories
Spaghetti, 1 cup, whole-wheat, cooked	1.2	145	174
Veal chop, 3.5 ounces, lean, roasted	1.8	97	175
Ham, 3.5 ounces, 11 percent fat	1.8	99	178
Steak, 3.5 ounces, select sirloin, broiled	1.8	100	180
Sautéed Flounder with Lemon Sauce, page 196	1.2	150	180
Fiesta Fish Stew, page 202	0.40	463	185
Turkey, 3.5 ounces, dark meat without skin	1.9	98	187
Vegetable pizza, 1 slice, ⅛ of 12-inch-diameter pie, regular crust	2.5	76	191
Chicken breast, 3.5 ounces, roasted, with skin	2.0	97	193
Meat-and-vegetable pizza, 1 slice, ⅛ of 12-inch-diameter pie, thin crust	2.4	80	193
Pork Chops with Orange-Soy Sauce, page 188	1.6	122	195
Turkey, 3.5 ounces, light meat with skin	2.0	98	195
Catfish, 3 ounces, battered and fried	2.3	85	195
Macaroni, 1 cup cooked	1.4	141	197
Spaghetti, 1 cup cooked	1.4	141	197

200 to 300 calories

	Energy Density	Weight (grams)	Calories
Tuna and White Bean Salad, page 150	0.66	303	200
Open-Faced Roast Beef Sandwich, page 118	1.1	182	200
Chicken Parmesan, page 205	1.8	111	200
Duck, 3.5 ounces, without skin	2.1	96	201
Lean pork chop, 3.5 ounces, center loin, broiled	2.0	101	202
Cheese pizza, 1 slice, ⅛ of 12-inch-diameter pie, thick crust	2.8	72	202
Meat pizza, 1 slice, ⅛ of 12-inch-diameter pie, thin crust	2.9	72	208
Poach-Roast Salmon with Yogurt and Dill Sauce, page 193	1.6	140	225
Turkey, 3.5 ounces dark meat with skin	2.2	100	219
Buffalo chicken wings, 3.5 ounces, with skin	2.3	100	229
Fillet of Sole and Vegetable Parcels, page 197	0.70	329	230
Turkey, 3.5 ounces, ground	2.4	97	233
Meat and vegetable pizza, 1 slice, ⅛ of 12-inch-diameter pie, thick crust	2.7	87	234
Goose, 3.5 ounces, without skin	2.4	99	238
Beef ravioli, 1 cup, canned in tomato and meat sauce	0.95	252	239
Chicken Merlot, page 206	0.70	343	240

	Energy Density	Weight (grams)	Calories
Meat pizza, 1 slice, ⅛ of 12-inch-diameter pie, thick crust	3.1	78	243
Nouveau Lamb Stew, page 186	0.40	613	245
Stir-Fried Beef with Snow Peas and Cherry Tomatoes, page 181	1.2	213	255
Thai Chicken Salad, page 142	0.71	359	255
Ground beef, 3.5 ounces, extra lean, broiled	2.6	98	256
Chicken breast, 3.5 ounces, with skin, breaded, fried	2.6	99	258
Pizza Margherita, page 239	1.3	204	265
Penne with Olives and Spinach, page 232	1.4	189	265
Classic Vegetarian Vegetable Stew, page 176	0.60	450	270
Ground beef, 3.5 ounces, lean, broiled	2.7	101	272
Almond Chicken Salad Sandwich, page 114	1.4	196	275
Swedish meatballs with pasta, 1 reduced-calorie frozen entrée, 9.1 ounces	1.1	251	276
California Cobb Salad, page 143	0.82	341	280
Zesty Tuna Salad Pita, page 124	1.2	238	285
Garden Fresh Vegetable Pizza, page 238	1.2	238	285
Manicotti with 3 cheeses, 1 reduced-calorie frozen entrée, 11 ounces	0.93	312	290
Risotto Primavera, page 222	1.0	290	290
The Aristotle Pizza, page 237	1.0	290	290
Roasted Portobello Sandwich, page 119	1.2	242	290
Turkey-Pepperoni Pizza, page 242	1.6	184	295
Cornish game hen, ½ bird, with skin	2.6	114	296
Chicken pieces, 3.5 ounces, boneless, breaded and fried	3.0	100	299

300 to 400 calories

	Energy Density	Weight (grams)	Calories
Bayou Red Beans and Rice, page 218	0.90	333	300
Mediterranean Turkey Sandwich, page 117	1.4	214	300
Asian Chicken Wraps, page 122	1.1	282	310
All American Hamburger, page 126	1.5	207	310
Garden Chili, page 216	0.70	450	315
Shepherd's Pie, page 184	0.90	350	315
South of the Border Chicken Stew, page 208	0.50	650	325
Chickpea Curry, page 174	0.70	464	325
Shrimp Fried Rice, page 200	1.1	295	325
Paella Sencillo, page 220	1.2	271	325

Energy	Weight Density	Calories (grams)	
Stir-Fried Turkey with Crunchy Vegetables, page 211	0.80	413	330
Veggie-Stuffed Macaroni and Cheese, page 234	1.0	330	330
Old World Goulash, page 182	0.60	558	335
Shrimp Creole, page 199	0.60	558	335
Duck, 3.5 ounces, with skin	3.4	99	337
Charlie's Pasta Primavera, page 228	0.80	431	345
Cold-Cut Combo Sandwich, page 116	1.2	288	345
Buffalo Chicken Wraps, page 120	1.2	292	350
Vegetarian lasagna, 1 cup	1.4	250	350
Eggplant "Lasagna," page 175	1.1	322	355
Mushroom and Cheese Quesadillas with Mango Salsa, page 85	1.4	214	355
Jenny's Caribbean Tuna and Fruit Kebobs, page 198	1.0	360	360
Pasta helper mix with cheese and ground beef, 1 cup	1.6	225	360
Broccoli and Tomato Stuffed Shells, page 236	1.0	370	370
Tofu Pad Thai, page 167	0.90	417	375
Chicken and Avocado Pita Pockets, page 123	1.3	288	375
Crisp Stir-Fried Vegetables, page 166	0.80	481	385
Chicken Fajita Pizza, page 240	1.6	244	390
Macaroni and cheese, 1 cup	2.0	196	392
Lasagna with meat, 1 cup	1.6	249	399

More than 400 calories

Santa Fe Steak Salad with Lime-Cilantro Dressing, page 144	0.79	506	400
Oceanside Pasta, page 230	0.80	500	400
Liz's Pasta Salad, page 146	0.82	488	400
Spaghetti with Tomato and Fresh Basil Sauce, page 233	1.0	400	400

Desserts Modular List

Dessert calories can add up quickly unless you choose those low in energy density or limit your portions. I have listed most fruit with the snacks, but fruit provides a nutritious and satisfying end to a meal.

	Energy Density	Weight (grams)	Calories
Less than 100 calories			
Fruit-flavored gelatin, ½ cup, sugar-free	0.07	143	10
Balsamic Berries, page 246	0.37	149	55
Vanilla pudding, ½ cup, sugar-free, prepared with nonfat milk	0.53	132	70
Frozen fruit and juice bar, 3 ounces	0.82	91	75
Chocolate pudding, ½ cup, sugar-free, prepared with nonfat milk	0.60	133	80
Fruit-flavored gelatin, ½ cup	0.59	141	83
Light vanilla ice cream, ½ cup	1.4	66	92
100 to 200 calories			
Baked apple, 1 medium item, unsweetened	0.63	162	102
Italian ice, 1 cup, lemon	0.53	232	123
Four-Fruit Compote, page 249	0.38	329	125
Ruby-Red Poached Pears with Raspberry Sauce, page 250	0.60	208	125
Maple Crème Caramel, page 258	1.0	130	130
Vanilla pudding, ½ cup, prepared with 2 percent milk	1.1	128	141
Fruit-flavored frozen yogurt, ½ cup	1.3	111	144
Chocolate pudding, ½ cup, prepared with 2 percent milk	1.1	136	150
Raspberry-Topped Ricotta Cakes, page 255	1.1	150	165
Fresh Fruit Parfait, page 252	0.78	218	170
Raspberry-Apple Crumble, page 254	1.0	175	175
Coffee cake with crumb topping, 1 slice, ⅛ of 8 inch cake	3.2	56	178
Grilled Banana Splits, page 248	1.2	154	185
Chocolate Fondue with Fresh Fruit, page 259	1.2	155	185
Chocolate snack cake, 1 cream-filled, frosted	3.6	52	188

	Energy Density	Weight (grams)	Calories
200 to 300 calories			
Rice pudding, ½ cup	1.4	155	217
Cherry pie, 1 slice, ⅛ of 9-inch frozen pie, reduced-fat, no sugar added	1.8	122	220
Pumpkin pie, 1 slice, ⅙ of 8-inch frozen pie	2.1	109	229
Strawberry Trifle with Lemon Cream, page 256	1.2	208	250
Brownie, 2-inch square	4.4	61	269
Ice cream, ½ cup, premium, vanilla/chocolate	2.5	108	270
More than 300 calories			
Banana cream pie, 1 slice, ⅛ of 9-inch pie	2.7	147	398
German chocolate cake with frosting, 1 slice, 1/12 of 9-inch cake	3.6	112	404
Apple pie, 1 slice, ⅛ of 9-inch pie	2.7	152	411
Cheese cake, 1 slice, ⅙ of 9-inch cake	3.6	127	457
Carrot cake with cream cheese frosting, 1 slice, 1/12 of 9-inch cake	4.4	110	484
Cherry pie, 1 slice, ⅛ of 9-inch pie	2.7	180	486

Snacks Modular List

The snacks modular list contains a wide variety of foods that can be eaten between meals. You will find raw vegetables, fruits, potato chips, cookies, and candy. You can also snack on foods from other lists, such as soup or cereal. Choose your snacks wisely! Although I have included foods high in energy density, they are not your best choices. They are too easy to overeat, and are less filling than foods low in energy density. Many of the foods in this section, such as fruit and yogurt, make nutritious desserts.

	Energy Density	Weight (grams)	Calories
Less than 100 calories			
Cucumber, ½ cup	0.13	77	10
Celery, 1 stalk	0.16	81	13
Bell peppers, ½ cup	0.27	74	20
Hard candy, 1 piece	3.9	6	24
Tomato, 1 medium	0.21	124	26
Rice cake, plain	3.9	9	35
Tangerine, 1 medium	0.44	84	37
Clementine, 1 medium	0.44	84	37
Canned fruit cocktail, in light syrup, ½ cup	0.31	119	38
Plum, 1 medium	0.61	66	40
Popsicle, 2-ounce bar	0.72	58	42
Peach, 1 medium	0.43	98	42
Strawberries, 1 cup	0.30	143	43
Kiwifruit, 1 medium	0.61	75	46
Mandarin oranges, canned, ½ cup	0.36	125	46
Olives, black, 10 each	1.1	46	51
Cantaloupe, 1 cup	0.35	160	56
Raspberries, 1 cup	0.48	123	60
Grapes, 1 cup	0.67	93	62
Honeydew, 1 cup	0.35	177	62
Orange, 1 medium	0.47	132	62
Dried apricots, ¼ cup	1.1	66	73
Angel-food cake, 1-ounce slice, approximately 1/12 cake	2.6	28	73
Grapefruit, 1 medium	0.30	247	74
Pineapple, 1 cup	0.49	155	76
Hard-boiled egg	1.6	49	78
B's Favorite Smoothie, page 90	0.42	190	80
Gelatin, ½ cup	0.59	136	80
String cheese, 1 ounce	2.8	29	80
Blueberries, 1 cup	0.56	145	81
Apple, 1 medium	0.58	140	81
Cottage cheese, 1 percent fat, ½ cup	0.73	122	82
Baby carrots, 15, with 1 tablespoon nonfat ranch dressing	0.53	155	82
Ice cream, nonfat, ½ cup	1.3	69	90

	Energy Density	Weight (grams)	Calories
Mel's Fresh Lemon Hummus, page 77	1.7	53	90
Fudgsicle, 1.75-ounce item	1.8	74	90
Vanilla wafers, 5 each	4.5	21	94
Pear, 1 medium	0.59	166	98

100 to 200 calories

	Energy Density	Weight (grams)	Calories
Nonfat chocolate pudding, 1 snack cup	0.88	113	100
Fat-free potato chips, 1 ounce	3.5	28	100
Orange sherbet, ½ cup	1.4	73	102
Ice cream, light, ½ cup	1.2	90	108
Banana, 1 medium	0.92	118	109
Raisins, ¼ cup	3.0	36	109
Fig cookies, Newton type, 2	3.5	31	110
Popcorn, air-popped, 1 ounce	3.8	28	110
Soy nuts, honey roasted, 1 ounce	3.9	28	110
Baked tortilla chips, 1 ounce	3.9	28	110
Baked potato chips, 1 ounce	3.9	28	110
Pound cake, 1-ounce slice	3.8	28	110
Granola bar, chewy, low-fat, 1 ounce	4.0	28	111
Animal crackers, 10	4.5	25	112
Pretzels, 1 ounce	3.9	29	113
Frozen yogurt, soft serve, ½ cup	1.6	71	114
Graham crackers, 4 each	4.2	28	118
Baked tortilla chips, 1 ounce, with ¼ cup salsa	2.0	60	119
Yogurt, nonfat, flavored with aspartame, 8 ounces	0.53	226	120
Fruit sorbet, ½ cup	1.1	109	120
Wheat bagel, 1 half 4" bagel, with 1 tablespoon light cream cheese	2.1	58	120
Rice cake, plain, with 1 tablespoon peanut butter	5.2	25	130
Trail mix, 1 ounce	4.7	28	131
Broth-based canned soup, 1 cup	0.51	261	133
Apple, ½, with 1 tablespoon peanut butter	1.6	85	135
Popcorn, oil-popped, 1 ounce	5.1	28	142
Regular tortilla chips, 1 ounce	5.1	28	142
Cheese, 1-ounce reduced-fat Cheddar with 7 thin wheat crackers	3.6	40	144
Regular potato chips, 1 ounce	5.4	28	152

	Energy Density	Weight (grams)	Calories
Corn chips, 1 ounce	5.4	28	153
Jelly beans, 15 large	3.7	42	156
Cheese puffs, 1 ounce	5.6	28	157
Chocolate pudding, 1 snack cup	1.4	113	160
Tropical Island Smoothie, page 91	0.70	236	165
Avocado, ½, with lemon juice	1.1	152	170
Sunflower seed kernels, ¼ cup, roasted, toasted	5.8	32	186
Mixed nuts, ¼ cup, dry roasted	5.8	33	190
More than 200 calories			
Almonds, ¼ cup, dry roasted	5.9	35	206
Soft pretzel, 2.25 ounces	3.5	62	215
Yogurt, low-fat, flavored, 8 ounces	1.0	220	220

Condiments Modular List

Remember to add the calories from toppings, spreads, and condiments when budgeting your calories. Notice how many calories the high-fat, energy-dense condiments like mayonnaise add to a dish.

	Energy Density	Weight (grams)	Calories
Less than 100 calories			
Vinegar, 1 tablespoon	0.14	14	2
Salsa, 1 tablespoon	0.32	16	5
Mayonnaise, 1 tablespoon, nonfat	0.62	16	10
Cherry Tomato Salsa, page 240	0.25	40	10
Mustard, 1 tablespoon	0.80	15	12
Barbecue sauce, 1 tablespoon	0.75	16	12
Cream cheese, 1 tablespoon, nonfat	0.95	15	14
Yogurt and Dill Sauce, page 193	0.52	29	15
Yogurt Cheese, page 89	0.90	17	15
Ketchup, 1 tablespoon	1.1	15	16
Raspberry Sauce, page 250	0.80	25	20
Soy-Ginger Dipping Sauce, page 82	1.2	21	25
Pancake syrup, 1 tablespoon, reduced-calorie	1.6	16	25
House Dressing, page 76	0.75	40	30
Dijon Vinaigrette, page 152	1.2	29	35
Cream cheese, 1 tablespoon, reduced fat	2.2	16	35
Lime-Cilantro Dressing, page 144	1.6	24	38
Marshmallow cream topping, 2 tablespoons	3.3	12	40
Orange-Poppy Seed Dressing, page 138	1.2	38	45
Balsamic Dressing, page 152	2.0	22	45
Marmalade, jelly, or preserves, 1 tablespoon	2.4	20	48
Mayonnaise, 1 tablespoon, reduced-fat	3.3	15	50
Margarine, 1 tablespoon, reduced-fat	3.5	14	50
Cream cheese, 1 tablespoon, full-fat	3.5	15	51
Maple syrup, 1 tablespoon	2.6	20	52
Pancake syrup, 1 tablespoon	2.9	20	57

	Energy Density	Weight (grams)	Calories
Mango Salsa, page 88	0.58	103	60
Honey, 1 tablespoon	3.0	21	64
Guacamole, page 88	0.83	78	65
Citrus-Ginger Dressing, page 153	3.1	21	65
Peanut butter, 1 tablespoon	5.9	16	94
Tex-Mex Salsa, page 78	0.65	146	95

100 to 200 calories

	Energy Density	Weight (grams)	Calories
Mayonnaise, 1 tablespoon	7.1	14	100
Almond butter, 1 tablespoon	6.3	16	101
Margarine, 1 tablespoon	7.2	14	101
Butter, 1 tablespoon	7.2	15	108
Fudge topping, 2 tablespoons	3.5	42	146

Beverages Modular List

You will notice that, with the exception of milk, beverages were not included in the menu plan. This does not mean that you are not allowed to have beverages; just make sure that you budget the calories. So, if you want a glass of wine with dinner, skip dessert or save some calories at snack time. Remember that beverage calories add to food calories, so substitute low-calorie or zero-calorie beverages whenever you can.

	Energy Density	Weight (grams)	Calories
Water, 8 fluid ounces	0.00	237	0
Club soda, 12 fluid ounces	0.00	360	0
Diet cola/soda, 12 fluid ounces	0.00	360	0
Tea, brewed, without sugar, 8 fluid ounces	0.10	237	2
Coffee, 8 fluid ounces	0.20	237	5
Vegetable juice, 8 fluid ounces	0.19	242	46
White wine, 4 fluid ounces	0.68	118	80
Orange juice, 6 fluid ounces	0.45	186	84
Red wine, 4 fluid ounces	0.72	118	85
Milk, nonfat, 8 fluid ounces	0.35	245	86
Apple juice, unsweetened, 6 fluid ounces	0.47	186	87
Light beer, 12 fluid ounces	0.28	354	99
Milk, low-fat (1 percent), 8 fluid ounces	0.42	244	102
Whiskey, 1.5 fluid ounces	2.5	42	104
Grape juice, 6 fluid ounces	0.61	186	113
Wine cooler, 8 fluid ounces	0.50	240	120
Milk, reduced-fat (2 percent), 8 fluid ounces	0.50	244	122
Beer, 12 fluid ounces	0.41	356	146
Milk, whole (3.3 percent), 8 fluid ounces	0.61	244	149
Chocolate soy milk, 8 fluid ounces	0.62	242	150
Cola/soda, 12 fluid ounces	0.41	372	152
Orange soda, 12 fluid ounces	0.46	360	167
Sherry, dry, 4 fluid ounces	1.4	120	168
Daiquiri, 4 fluid ounces	1.9	121	224
Margarita, 4 fluid ounces	2.2	124	271
Eggnog, 8 fluid ounces	1.4	245	343

Resources

5 A DAY and Produce for Better Health Foundation

Are you eating at least five servings of fruits and vegetables each day? Want to learn why you should and how you do it? Visit the Produce for Better Health Foundation's website, http://www.5aday.org. It contains tips, recipes, and health information. This campaign is also featured on the National Cancer Institute's website, www.5aday.gov, which provides even more information to help you eat a healthier diet.

American Dietetic Association

This is the website of the largest association for nutrition professionals in the United States. If you are interested in nutrition counseling, there are resources listed to help you find a Registered Dietitian (R.D.) in your area. To speak with someone on the Consumer Nutrition Hot Line, call 1-800-366-1655 from 8 A.M. to 5 P.M., Central Standard Time. Website: www.eatright.org.

American Institute for Cancer Research

The American Institute for Cancer Research funds research and provides consumer information on the link between diet and cancer. A quarterly newsletter gives an update on current research and offers food preparation tips to maximize the healthiness of your diet. Make sure you check out *The New American Plate* and the *Recipe Corner* sections to get tips and a wide range of healthy recipes that taste good. Website: www.aicr.org.

America on the Move

Are you having difficulty staying motivated to exercise? America on the Move may be the website for you. It is a national program dedicated to helping individuals and communities make positive changes to achieve healthy eating and active living habits. Registration is free and will give you access to tips for healthy eating and activity, as well as letting you enter your daily step count as a way to monitor your progress. Opportunities are also available for you to organize a walking group in your community. Website: http://www.americaonthemove.org/

Center for Nutrition Policy and Promotion (US Department of Agriculture)

The *Consumer Corner,* linked with the Food and Nutrition Information Center, contains information about food and nutrition topics that most consumers want to know. In addition to answers to frequently asked questions, this site has tips on cooking, recipes, and links to other resources. Website: http://www.nal.usda.gov/fnic/consumersite/

Center for Science in the Public Interest (CSPI)

CSPI is a nonprofit consumer advocacy group with a strong focus on nutrition. They publish the *Nutrition Action Healthletter.* They offer information about the most up-to-date nutrition topics. Website: www.cspinet.org

Delicious Decisions (American Heart Association)

Provided by the American Heart Association, this website offers information on healthy food shopping, cooking, and dining out. In addition, over 200 heart-healthy recipes are available. Website: http://www.deliciousdecisions.org/

Fitness.gov

Want to learn more about physical activity and fitness? Check out this website designed by The President's Council on Physical Fitness and Sports, http://

www.fitness.gov/. You will also find a link to the President's Challenge website, http://www.presidentschallenge.org/. This website provides information on how to increase your daily activity and allows you to monitor your progress. Registration is required, but is free.

Health-e-Weight for Women

This comprehensive site emphasizes healthful eating, which includes information on weight management. The articles cover nutrition basics, tips for easy shopping, the importance of exercise, and long-term strategies for weight maintenance. Interactive tools, such as body-mass index, physical activity, and waist-to-hip ratio calculators can help you determine and monitor your goals. Website: http://www.brighamandwomens.org/healtheweightforwomen/

The International Food Information Council (IFIC)

This food-industry sponsored site provides scientific information on a wide variety of topics about nutrition and food safety. Website: www.ific.org

Nutrition and Physical Activity (Centers for Disease Control—CDC)

The CDC has put together a website that has information on current topics related to nutrition, physical activity, and overall health. Click on all of the links to find substantial information about health-related topics. Website: http://www.cdc.gov/nccdphp/dnpa/

Nutrition.gov

Are you interested in learning more about the nutritional quality of the food you eat? Check out Nutrition.gov at http://www.nutrition.gov/home/index.php3. This site has access to the USDA National Nutrient Database, on which you can search for nutritional information on specific foods. This site also has information on nutrition, food safety, and health management.

Shape Up America

Former Surgeon General C. Everett Koop started this campaign to reduce obesity and increase fitness. This site has up-to-date information on weight management, healthy eating, and physical fitness. It helps you to develop a fun and effective activity program. Website: www.shapeup.org

Small steps.gov (US Department of Health and Human Services)

Like America on the Move, Fitness.gov, and Shape Up America, this website offers suggestions as to how to increase your activity and monitor your progress. They also have a newsletter that gives tips, recipes, and more. Website: http://www.smallstep.gov/

Tufts University Nutrition Navigator

Not finding the right website on this list, or would you just like to visit other nutrition-related websites to learn more? Go to the Tufts University website: www.navigator.tufts.edu. Tufts' nutritionists review and rate the quality and ease of use of hundreds of nutrition-related websites.

Weight Loss and Control (National Institutes of Health: NIDDK)

Developed by the National Institutes of Diabetes & Digestive & Kidney diseases, this website has a list of links to information about weight loss and weight management. Website: http://www.niddk.nih.gov/health/nutrit/nutrit.htm. It also has a link to the Weight-control Information Network (WINS), which was designed to provide scientific information to the public about weight management. WINS also has a free quarterly newsletter that you can sign up for.

References

Anderson, G. H. and Moore, S. E. (2004). Dietary proteins in the regulation of food intake and body weight in humans. *Journal of Nutrition*, 134, 947S–979S.

Anderson, G. H. and Woodend, D. (2003). Consumption of sugars and the regulation of short-term satiety and food intake. *American Journal of Clinical Nutrition*, 78 (suppl), 843S–849S.

Bell, E. A., Castellanos, V. H., Pelkman, C. L., Thorwart, M. L. and Rolls, B. J. (1998). Energy density of foods affects energy intake in normal-weight women. *American Journal of Clinical Nutrition*, 67, 412–420.

Caton, S. J., Ball, M., Ahern, A. and Hetherington, M. M. (2004). Dose-dependent effects of alcohol on appetite and food intake. *Physiology and Behavior*, 81, 51–58.

Diliberti, N., Bordi, P., Conklin, M. T., Roe, L. S. and Rolls, B. J. (2004). Increased portion size leads to increased energy intake in a restaurant meal. *Obesity Research*, 12, 562–568.

Eisenstein, J., Roberts, S. B., Dallal, G. and Saltzman, E. (2002). High-protein weight-loss diets: are they safe and do they work? A review of the experimental and epidemiologic data. *Nutrition Reviews*, 60, 189–200.

Feinle, C., O'Donovan, D. and Horowitz, M. (2002). Carbohydrate and satiety. *Nutrition Reviews*, 60, 155–169.

First Data Bank, Inc. (2004). Nutritionist Pro (computer software). San Bruno, CA.

Howarth, N. C., Saltzman, E. and Roberts, S. B. (2001). Dietary fiber and weight regulation. *Nutrition Reviews*, 59, 129–139.

Institute of Medicine of the National Academies (2002). *Dietary Reference Intakes: Energy, Carbohydrate, Fiber, Fat, Fatty Acids, Cholesterol, Protein, and Amino Acids*. Washington, D. C.: The National Academies Press.

Jakicic, J. M., Marcus, B. H., Gallagher, K. L., Napolitano, M. and Lang, W. (2003). Effect of exercise duration and intensity on weight loss in overweight, sedentary women. *JAMA: The Journal of the American Medical Association*, 290, 1323–1330.

Klein, S., Sheard, N. F., Pi-Sunyer, X., Daly, A., Wylie-Rosett, J., Kulkarni, K. and Clark, N. G. (2004). Weight management through lifestyle modification for the prevention and management of type 2 diabetes: rationale and strategies. A statement of the American Diabetes Association, the North American Association for the Study of Obesity, and the American Society for Clinical Nutrition. *American Journal of Clinical Nutrition, 80*, 257–263.

Klem, M. L., Wing, R. R., Lang, W., McGuire, M. T. and Hill, J. O. (2000). Does weight loss maintenance become easier over time? *Obesity Research, 8*, 438–444.

Koh-Banerjee, P. and Rimm, E. B. (2003). Whole grain consumption and weight gain: a review of the epidemiological evidence, potential mechanisms and opportunities for future research. *Proceedings of the Nutrition Society, 62*, 25–29.

Kral, T. V. E., Roe, L. S. and Rolls, B. J. (2004). Combined effects of energy density and portion size on energy intake in women. *American Journal of Clinical Nutrition, 79*, 962–968.

Liu, S., Willett, W. C., Manson, J. E., Hu, F. B., Rosner, B. and Colditz, G. A. (2003). Relation between changes in intakes of dietary fiber and grain products and changes in weight and development of obesity among middle-aged women. *American Journal of Clinical Nutrition, 78*, 920–927.

National Institutes of Health (1998). National Heart, Lung, and Blood Institute. *Clinical Guidelines on the Identification, Evaluation, and Treatment of Overweight and Obesity in Adults.* Washington, DC: U.S. Department of Health and Human Services.

Pennington, J. A. T. and Douglass, J. S. (2005). *Bowes & Church's Food Values of Portions Commonly Used.* 18th Edition. Baltimore: Lippincott, Williams & Wilkins.

Poppitt, S. D. (1995). Energy density of diets and obesity. *International Journal of Obesity, 19*, S20–S26.

Prentice, A. M. and Jebb, S. A. (2003). Fast foods, energy density and obesity: a possible mechanistic link. *Obesity Reviews, 4*, 187–194.

Rolls, B. J. (1985). Experimental analyses of the effects of variety in a meal on human feeding. *American Journal of Clinical Nutrition, 42*, 932–939.

Rolls, B. J. (2003). The supersizing of America: portion size and the obesity epidemic. *Nutrition Today, 38*, 42–53.

Rolls, B. J. and Barnett, R. A. (2000). *The Volumetrics Weight-Control Plan.* New York: Quill, 2000.

Rolls, B. J. and Bell, E. A. (2000). Dietary approaches to the treatment of obesity. In M. D. Jensen (ed.), *Medical Clinics of North America* (Vol. 84, March 2000, pp. 401–418). Philadelphia: W. B. Saunders Company.

Rolls, B. J., Bell, E. A. and Thorwart, M. L. (1999). Water incorporated into a food but not served with a food decreases energy intake in lean women. *American Journal of Clinical Nutrition,* 70, 448–455.

Rolls, B. J., Castellanos, V. H., Halford, J. C., Kilara, A., Panyam, D., Pelkman, C. L., Smith, G. P. and Thorwart, M. L. (1998). Volume of food consumed affects satiety in men. *American Journal of Clinical Nutrition,* 67, 1170–1177.

Rolls, B. J., Ello-Martin, J. A. and Tohill, B. C. (2004). What can intervention studies tell us about the relationship between fruit and vegetable consumption and weight management? *Nutrition Reviews,* 62, 1–17.

Rolls, B. J. and Hill, J. O. (1998) *Carbohydrates and weight management.* ILSI Press Washington, D.C.

Rolls, B. J., Roe, L. S., Kral, T. V. E., Meengs, J. S. and Wall, D. E. (2004). Increasing the portion size of a packaged snack increases energy intake in men and women. *Appetite,* 42, 63–69.

Rolls, B. J., Roe, L. S., Meengs, J. S. and Wall, D. E. (2004). Increasing the portion size of a sandwich increases energy intake. *Journal of the American Dietetic Association,* 104, 367–372.

Rolls, B. J., Roe, L. S. and Meengs, J. S. (2004). Salad and satiety: energy density and portion size of a first course salad affect energy intake at lunch. *Journal of the American Dietetic Association,* 104, 1570–1576.

St. Jeor, S. T., Howard, B. V., Prewitt, E., Bovee, V., Bazzarre, T. and Eckel, R. H. (2001). Dietary protein and weight reduction. A statement for healthcare professionals from the Nutrition Committee of the Council on Nutrition, Physical Activity, and Metabolism of the American Heart Association. *Circulation,* 104, 1869–1874.

Saris, W. H. M. (2003). Sugars, energy metabolism, and body weight control. *American Journal of Clinical Nutrition,* 78 (suppl), 850S–857S.

Slentz, C. A., Duscha, B. D., Johnson, J. L., Ketchum, K., Aiken, L. B., Samsa, G. P., et al. (2004). Effects of the amount of exercise on body weight, body composition, and measures of central obesity: STRRIDE—a randomized controlled study. *Archives of Internal Medicine,* 164, 31–39.

Stubbs, R. J., Johnstone, A. M., O'Reilly, L. M., Barton, K. and Reid, C. (1998). The effect of covertly manipulating the energy density of mixed diets on ad libitum food intake in 'pseudo free-living' humans. *International Journal of Obesity,* 22, 980–987.

Swinburn, B. A., Caterson, I., Seidell, J. C. and James, W. P. T. (2004). Diet, nutrition and the prevention of excess weight gain and obesity. *Public Health Nutrition, 7,* 123–146.

Wing, R. R. and Hill, J. O. (2001). Successful weight loss maintenance. *Annual Review of Nutrition, 21,* 323–341.

Wyatt, H. R., Grunwald, G. K., Mosca, C. L., Klem, M. L., Wing, R. R. and Hill, J. O. (2002). Long-term weight loss and breakfast in subjects in the National Weight Control Registry. *Obesity Research, 10,* 78–82.

Yao, M. and Roberts, S. B. (2001). Dietary energy density and weight regulation. *Nutrition Reviews, 59,* 247–258.

Index

A

aerobic activity, 44
alcoholic beverages:
    calories in, 9, 21, 24, 25
    in weight management, 29
All American Hamburger, 126
Almond Chicken Salad Sandwich, 114–15
America on the Move, 47
appetizers and snacks, 71–91
    Asian Spring Rolls with Soy-Ginger
        Dipping Sauce, 82–83
    B's Favorite Smoothie, 90
    Guacamole, 88
    House Dressing, 76
    Insalata Caprese, 81
    Lemon Shrimp Bruschetta, 80
    Mango Salsa, 88
    Mel's Fresh Lemon Hummus, 77
    modular food list, 286–89
    Mushroom and Cheese Quesadillas
        with Mango Salsa, 85
    Sesame Mushroom Kebobs, 84
    Stuffed Mushrooms Florentine, 86–87
    Tex-Mex Salsa, 78
    Tropical Island Smoothie, 91
    Vegetable Party Platter, 74–75
    White Bean Bruschetta, 79
    Yogurt Cheese, 89

Apple-Raspberry Crumble, 254
Applesauce Muffins, Blueberry, 68
Apricot Oatmeal, Creamy, 69
Aristotle Pizza, The, 237
Arugula, Fennel, and Orange Salad, 133
Asian Black Bean Soup, 104
Asian Chicken Wraps, 122
Asian Spring Rolls with Soy-Ginger
        Dipping Sauce, 82–83
Asparagus, Roasted, 162
Autumn Harvest Pumpkin Soup, 96–97
avocados:
    California Cobb Salad with Nonfat
        Tomato and Herb Dressing, 143
    and Chicken Pita Pockets, 123
    Guacamole, 88

B

Baked Berry French Toast, 64
Baked Tilapia with Sautéed Vegetables,
    194–95
Balsamic Berries, 246–47
Balsamic Dressing, 152
Banana Splits, Grilled, 248
Barley:
    Herbed Stuffed Squash, 171
    Vegetarian Soup, 107

Basil, Fresh, Sauce, Spaghetti with
    Tomato and, 233
Bayou Red Beans and Rice, 218–19
beans, 213–14
    Black, Asian Soup, 104
    Cannellini, Soup, 105
    Chicken Fajita Pizza, 240–41
    Garden Chili, 216–17
    Green, Potato Salad with Tarragon
        and, 149
    Green, Stir-Fried, 164–65
    Red, Bayou Rice and, 218–19
    White Bean and Tuna Salad, 150–51
    White Bean Bruschetta, 79
beef:
    Garden Chili, 216–17
    Old World Goulash, 182–83
    Santa Fe Steak Salad with Lime-
        Cilantro Dressing, 144–45
    Shepherd's Pie, 184–85
    Stir-Fried, with Snow Peas and
        Tomatoes, 181
beer, 24
berries:
    Baked Berry French Toast, 64
    Balsamic, 246–47
    see also fruits
beverages, 9, 21, 24, 25
    modular list, 292
    in personal eating plan, 264
Black Bean Soup, Asian, 104
Blueberry Applesauce Muffins, 68
body-mass index (BMI), 34–36
breadcrumbs, 175

breakfast, 59–69
    Baked Berry French Toast, 64
    Blueberry Applesauce Muffins, 68
    calcium in, 60
    cereals, 60
    Creamy Apricot Oatmeal, 69
    fruit, 61
    Jennifer's Fruit-Smothered Whole-
        Wheat Buttermilk Pancakes,
        62–63
    Mexican Egg Wrap, 65
    modular food list, 273–75
    Piquant Frittata, 66–67
    protein in, 61
Broccoli:
    Creamy Soup, 98–99
    Minted, 158–59
    and Tomato Stuffed Shells, 236
Bruschetta:
    Lemon Shrimp, 80
    White Bean, 79
B's Favorite Smoothie, 90
Buffalo Chicken Wraps, 120–21
bulgur, 215
    in Tabbouleh, 148
    and Vegetable Stuffed Peppers,
        172–73

C

calcium, 60, 264–65
California Cobb Salad with Nonfat
        Tomato and Herb Dressing, 143

calories:
 achieving your goal for, 263
 in beverages, 9, 21, 24, 25
 burning via exercise, 44
 calculating daily needs of, 36–43
 counting, 27–28
 definitions of, 19, 27
 eating fewer, 6, 8
 from fat, 9, 14
 in fiber, 9, 11–12
 in food groups, 9
 and food labels, 14
 tips on how to save, 28
 in weight management, 27–28, 29
calories per gram (energy density),
  8–11, 16–19
 calculating, 18–19
 categories of, 17, 22–23
 estimating, 20
 and fat, 8–9, 14
 and fiber, 11–12
 and food choices, 16–18
 in food labels, 7
 foods low in, 7
 and fruit, 244
 learning about, 39
 and nutrition facts label, 18–21
 and portion size, 25–26
 in protein-rich foods, 13
 and satiety, 8
Cannellini Bean Soup, 105
carbohydrates:
 calories in, 9
 energy density of, 9
 foods rich in, 11
 as fuel, 11–12
 and satiety, 11
 in weight management, 29
Category 1 foods, 17, 22
Category 2 foods, 17, 22
Category 3 foods, 17, 23
Category 4 foods, 17, 23
Cauliflower Soup, Curried, 100
cereals, 60
Charlie's Greek Salad, 130–31
Charlie's Pasta Primavera, 228–29
cheese:
 low or nonfat, 226, 227
 in salads, 129
 in sandwiches, 112
 Veggie-Stuffed Macaroni and, 234–35
 Yogurt, 89
cheesecakes, Raspberry-Topped Ricotta
  Cakes, 255
Cherry Tomato Salsa, 240
chicken:
 Almond Salad Sandwich, 114–15
 Asian Wraps, 122
 and Avocado Pita Pockets, 123
 Buffalo Wraps, 120–21
 California Cobb Salad with Nonfat
  Tomato and Herb Dressing, 143
 cooked breast meat, 114
 Fajita Pizza, 240–41
 Merlot, 206–7
 Paella Sencillo, 220
 Parmesan, 205
 Provençal, 210

chicken (*cont.*)

    South of the Border Stew, 208–9

    Thai Salad, 142

    and Vegetable Soup, Hearty, 108–9

Chickpea Curry, 174

Chili, Garden, 216–17

Chocolate Fondue with Fresh Fruit, 259

cholesterol, 14, 192

Chowder, Corn and Tomato, 95

Cilantro-Lime Dressing, 144–45

Citrus-Ginger Dressing, 153

Classic Vegetarian Vegetable Stew,
    176–77

Cobb Salad, California, with Nonfat
    Tomato and Herb Dressing, 143

Cobo, Pam, 31–32

coffee, 21

cola/soda, 24

Cold-Cut Combo Sandwich, 116

Cole Slaw:

    Pepper, 140–41

    Tangy, 139

Compote, Four-Fruit, 249

condiments modular list, 290–91

conversion chart, 301

Corn and Tomato Chowder, 95

Creamy Apricot Oatmeal, 69

Creamy Broccoli Soup, 98–99

Creamy Cucumber and Dill Salad,
    132

Crème Caramel, Maple, 258

Creole Shrimp, 199

Crisp Stir-Fried Vegetables, 166

Crumble, Raspberry-Apple, 254

Cucumber and Dill Salad, Creamy,
    132

cue control, 49

Curried Cauliflower Soup, 100

Curry, Chickpea, 174

D

daily energy requirements, 42, 43

daily self-monitoring form, 50–55, 57

desserts, 243–59

    Balsamic Berries, 246–47

    Chocolate Fondue with Fresh Fruit,
        259

    Four-Fruit Compote, 249

    Fresh Fruit Parfait, 252–53

    Grilled Banana Splits, 248

    Maple Crème Caramel, 258

    modular food list, 285–86

    Raspberry-Apple Crumble, 254

    Raspberry-Topped Ricotta Cakes,
        255

    Ruby-Red Poached Pears with
        Raspberry Sauce, 250–51

    Strawberry Trifle with Lemon Cream,
        256–57

dieting, 2, 6

Dijon Vinaigrette, 152

Dill:

    and Cucumber Salad, Creamy, 132

    and Yogurt Sauce, 193

dough, pizza wheat, 257

dressings, *see* salad dressings; salads

E

eating plan, 261–92
  beverages, 264
  calcium, 264–65
  calorie goal in, 263
  lifetime of, 266–67
  make your own, 262–64
  modular food lists, 273–92
  salt, 265
  summary, 268
  tips to save money, 266
  tools for, 2–3
  variety and affordability,
    265
  Week 1, 269
  Week 2, 270
  Week 3, 271
  Week 4 (blank), 272
Eggplant "Lasagna," 175
Egg Wrap, Mexican, 65
energy density, 8–11, 16–19
  calculating, 18–19
  categories of, 17, 22–23
  estimating, 20
  and fat, 8–9, 14
  and fiber, 11–12
  and food choices, 16–18
  in food labels, 7
  foods low in, 7
  and fruit, 244
  learning about, 39
  and nutrition facts label, 18–21
  and portion size, 25–26
  in protein-rich foods, 13
  and satiety, 8
  and water, 9
energy requirements:
  for men, 43
  for women, 42
exercise:
  burning calories via, 44
  see also physical activity

F

Fajita, Chicken, Pizza,
    240–41
fat, 13–16
  calories from, 9, 14
  and cholesterol, 14
  daily intake of, 14
  and energy density, 8–9, 14
  in fish and shellfish, 191
  foods with reduced content of,
    14
  grams per serving, 14
  healthy types of, 13, 14
  in meats, 180
  monounsaturated, 14
  and packaging claims, 14
  in partially hydrogenated oils, 14
  reduced intake of, 7, 29
  in salad dressings, 128, 129
  saturated, 14
  tips for reducing, 15
  transfats, 14

fennel:
    Lemony Salad, 136
    Orange, and Arugula Salad, 133
    Tabbouleh, 148
fiber:
    calories in, 9, 11–12
    and carbohydrates, 11
    and energy density, 11–12
    foods high in, 7, 11
    recommended daily intake of, 11
    and satiety, 11
    sources of, 12
    and weight management, 11–12, 29
    in whole foods, 12
Fiesta Fish Stew, 202
Fillet of Sole and Vegetable Parcels, 197
fish and shellfish, 191–202
    Baked Tilapia with Sautéed
      Vegetables, 194–95
    fat content of, 191
    Fiesta Fish Stew, 202
    Fillet of Sole and Vegetable Parcels, 197
    Jenny's Caribbean Tuna and Fruit
      Kebobs, 198
    main dish modular food list, 280–84
    mercury contamination of, 192
    Oceanside Pasta, 230–31
    omega-3 fatty acids in, 14, 191
    Paella Sencillo, 220
    Poach-Roast Salmon with Yogurt and
      Dill Sauce, 193
    in sandwiches, 113
    Sautéed Flounder with Lemon Sauce,
      196

    Shrimp Creole, 199
    Shrimp Fried Rice, 200–201
Florentine Stuffed Mushrooms, 86–87
Flounder, Sautéed, with Lemon Sauce,
    196
Fondue, Chocolate, with Fresh Fruit, 259
food choices, and energy density, 16–18
food diary, 37, 38, 39
food labels:
    and calories, 14
    and energy density, 18
    nutrition facts on, 14
    and satiety, 7
Four-Fruit Compote, 249
French Toast, Baked Berry, 64
Fresh Fruit:
    Chocolate Fondue with, 259
    Parfait, 252–53
    and Spinach Salad with Orange-
      Poppy Seed Dressing, 138
Fried Rice, Shrimp, 200–201
Frittata, Piquant, 66–67
fruits:
    Baked Berry French Toast, 64
    Balsamic Berries, 246–47
    for breakfast, 61
    for dessert, 243–59
    energy density in, 244
    fiber in, 11
    Four-Fruit Compote, 249
    Fresh, and Spinach Salad with
      Orange-Poppy Seed Dressing, 138
    Fresh, Chocolate Fondue with, 259
    Fresh, Parfait, 252–53

Grilled Banana Splits, 248
modular food list, 286–89
Raspberry-Apple Crumble, 254
Raspberry-Topped Ricotta Cakes,
   255
Ruby-Red Poached Pears with
   Raspberry Sauce, 250–51
in salads, 129
-Smothered Whole-Wheat
   Buttermilk Pancakes, Jennifer's,
   62–63
Strawberry Trifle with Lemon Cream,
   256–57
tips for adding to your diet, 244–45
whole, vs. juice, 12
fuel:
   calories as, 27
   carbohydrates as, 11–12
fullness and hunger, cycle of, 40

grains, 215
   Bulgur and Vegetable Stuffed
      Peppers, 172–73
   fiber in, 11, 12
   Herbed Barley Stuffed Squash, 171
   Mary's Quinoa with Lime, 224
   side dish modular food list, 278–80
   Tabbouleh, 148
   Vegetarian Barley Soup, 107
   whole, 12, 111
grams, defined, 19
Greek Salad, Charlie's, 130–31
Green Beans:
   Potato Salad with Tarragon and, 149
   Stir-Fried, 164–65
Gremolata, Roasted Lamb Chops with,
   190
Grilled Banana Splits, 248
Guacamole, 88

G

garam masala, 174
Garden Chili, 216–17
Garden-Fresh Vegetable Pizza, 238
Garlic-Roasted Vegetables, 160–61
Gazpacho, 110
Ginger:
   -Citrus Dressing, 153
   -Soy Dipping Sauce, 82–83
goals, personal, 32–34
goals chart, 33
Goulash, Old World, 182–83

H

ham, in Liz's Pasta Salad, 146–47
hamburgers:
   All American, 126
   fat in, 180
Hearty Chicken and Vegetable Soup,
   108–9
herbs:
   Herbed Barley Stuffed Squash, 171
   with pasta, 226
   in sandwiches, 113
   and Tomato Dressing, Nonfat, 143

House Dressing, 76
hummus:
  Mel's Fresh Lemon, 77
  in sandwiches, 113
hunger:
  cycle of fullness and, 40
  feelings of, 40

I

Insalata Caprese, 81
Insalata Mista, 137
Italian Dressing, 153
Italian Hero Cold-Cut Combo
    Sandwich, 116
Italian Turkey Spirals, 212

J

Jennifer's Fruit-Smothered Whole-
    Wheat Buttermilk Pancakes, 62–63
Jenny's Caribbean Tuna and Fruit
    Kebobs, 198
juice, 12, 24

K

Kebobs:
  Jenny's Caribbean Tuna and Fruit,
    198
  Sesame Mushroom, 84

L

Lamb Chops, Roasted, with Gremolata,
    190
Lamb Stew, Nouveau, 186–87
"Lasagna," Eggplant, 175
legumes, 213–14
Lehman, Dan and Ann, 265
Lemon Cream, Strawberry Trifle, 256–57
Lemon Sauce, Sautéed Flounder with,
    196
Lemon Shrimp Bruschetta, 80
Lemony Fennel Salad, 136
Lentil and Tomato Soup, 106
Lime-Cilantro Dressing, 144–45
Liz's Pasta Salad, 146–47

M

Macaroni and Cheese, Veggie-Stuffed,
    234–35
main dish modular food list, 280–84
Mango Salsa, 88
  Mushroom and Cheese Quesadillas
    with, 85
Maple Crème Caramel, 258
Margherita Pizza, 239
Mary's Quinoa with Lime, 224
meats, 179–90
  All American Hamburger, 126
  fat in, 180
  main dish modular food list, 280–84
  Nouveau Lamb Stew, 186–87

Old World Goulash, 182–83
Pork Chops with Orange-Soy Sauce,
    188–89
protein in, 179–80
Roast Beef Open-Faced Sandwich, 118
Roasted Lamb Chops with Gremolata,
    190
in sandwiches, 112
Santa Fe Steak Salad with Lime-
    Cilantro Dressing, 144–45
Shepherd's Pie, 184–85
Stir-Fried Beef with Snow Peas and
    Tomatoes, 181
Mediterranean Turkey Sandwich, 117
Mel's Fresh Lemon Hummus, 77
men, energy requirements for, 43
menu plan, 49, 261–91
metric conversion chart, 301
Mexican Egg Wrap, 65
milk, 24
Minestrone, 102–3
Minted Broccoli, 158–59
modular food lists, 273–92
    beverages, 292
    breakfast food, 273–75
    condiments, 290–91
    desserts, 285–86
    main dish, 280–84
    side dishes, 278–80
    snacks, 286–89
    soup, 276–77
money-saving tips, 266
monounsaturated fat, 14
Muffins, Blueberry Applesauce, 68

muscle, building, 44
mushrooms, 157
    and Cheese Quesadillas with Mango
        Salsa, 85
    Roasted Portobello Sandwich, 119
    in sandwiches, 112
    Sesame Kebobs, 84
    Stuffed Florentine, 86–87

N

New Potatoes with Peas, 168
Nonfat Tomato and Herb Dressing, 143
Nouveau Lamb Stew, 186–87
nutrients, as fuel, 6
Nutrition Facts label, 14, 18–21

O

Oatmeal, Creamy Apricot, 69
obesigenic environment, 1
obesity, 1, 2, 6
Oceanside Pasta, 230–31
Old World Goulash, 182–83
omega-3 fatty acids, 14, 191
O'Nan, Jill, 5
Open-Faced Roast Beef Sandwich, 118
Orange:
    Fennel, and Arugula Salad, 133
    –Poppy Seed Dressing, 138
    -Soy Sauce, Pork Chops with, 188–89
Oven-Roasted Potatoes, 169

P

Pad Thai, Tofu, 167
Paella Sencillo, 220
Pancakes, Jennifer's Fruit-Smothered
    Whole-Wheat Buttermilk, 62–63
Parfait, Fresh Fruit, 252–53
partially hydrogenated oils, 14
Party Vegetable Platter, 74–75
pasta, 225–36
    Broccoli and Tomato Stuffed Shells,
        236
    Liz's Salad, 146–47
    Oceanside, 230–31
    Penne with Olives and Spinach, 232
    Primavera, Charlie's, 228–29
    Spaghetti with Tomato and Fresh
        Basil Sauce, 233
    Veggie-Stuffed Macaroni and Cheese,
        234–35
Pears, Ruby-Red Poached, with
    Raspberry Sauce, 250–51
Peas, New Potatoes with, 168
pedometer, 45
Penne with Olives and Spinach, 232
Peppers, Bulgur and Vegetable Stuffed,
    172–73
Pepper Slaw, 140–41
personal eating plan, 261–92
    beverages, 264
    calcium, 264–65
    calorie goal for, 263
    customizing, 262–64
    for a lifetime, 266–67

modular food lists, 273–92
    salt, 265
    summary, 268
    tips to save money, 266
    variety and affordability, 265
    Week 1 menu, 269
    Week 2 menu, 270
    Week 3 menu, 271
    Week 4 (blank), 272
personal goals:
    for physical activity, 44–48
    and self-monitoring, 51
    and setting habits, 48–49
    tracking of, 32–34, 41
physical activity:
    aerobic, 44
    counting steps, 44–48
    goals for, 44–48
    muscle built in, 44
    in weight management, 29
Pilaf, Vegetable, 221
Piquant Frittata, 66–67
pizza, 226–27
    The Aristotle, 237
    calorie count in, 227
    Chicken Fajita, 240–41
    dough, wheat, 257
    Garden-Fresh Vegetable, 238
    Margherita, 239
    Turkey-Pepperoni, 242
plateaus, 52
Poach-Roast Salmon with Yogurt and
    Dill Sauce, 193
Poppy Seed-Orange Dressing, 138

Pork Chops with Orange-Soy Sauce, 188–89

portion control, 25–27, 226, 243

Portobello Sandwich, Roasted, 119

potatoes:

New, with Peas, 168

Oven-Roasted, 169

Salad with Green Beans and Tarragon, 149

Shepherd's Pie, 184–85

Smashed, 170

poultry, 203–12

Chicken Merlot, 206–7

Chicken Parmesan, 205

Chicken Provençal, 210

choosing, 203–4

Italian Turkey Spirals, 212

main dish modular food list, 280–84

Mediterranean Turkey Sandwich, 117

South of the Border Chicken Stew, 208–9

Stir-Fried Turkey with Crunchy Vegetables, 211

preventative eating, 157

protein:

for breakfast, 61

calories in, 9

energy density of, 9

food choice tips, 13

lean, 7

in meats, 179–80

in pasta sauces, 226

in pizza, 227

in salads, 129

and satiety, 13

in weight management, 12–13, 29, 179

Pumpkin Soup, Autumn Harvest, 96–97

Q

Quesadillas, Mushroom and Cheese, with Mango Salsa, 85

Quinoa with Lime, Mary's, 224

R

Raspberry:

-Apple Crumble, 254

Sauce, Ruby-Red Poached Pears with, 250–51

-Topped Ricotta Cakes, 255

Ratatouille, 162

Red Beans and Rice, Bayou, 218–19

resources, 293–96

rice, 214–15

Bayou Red Beans and, 218–19

Paella Sencillo, 220

Risotto Primavera, 222–23

Shrimp Fried, 200–201

Vegetable Pilaf, 221

Ricotta Cakes, Raspberry-Topped, 255

Risotto Primavera, 222–23

Roast Beef Open-Faced Sandwich, 118

Roasted Asparagus, 162

Roasted Lamb Chops with Gremolata, 190

Roasted Portobello Sandwich, 119
Ruby-Red Poached Pears with
    Raspberry Sauce, 250–51
Rustic Tomato Soup, 101

S

salad dressings:
    Balsamic, 152
    Citrus-Ginger, 153
    condiments modular list, 290–91
    Dijon Vinaigrette, 152
    and fat, 128, 129
    House, 76
    Italian, 153
    Lime-Cilantro, 144–45
    Nonfat Tomato and Herb, 143
    Orange-Poppy Seed, 138
    in sandwiches, 112–13
    see also salads
salads, 127–51
    Almond Chicken Sandwich, 114–15
    California Cobb, with Nonfat Tomato
        and Herb Dressing, 143
    Charlie's Greek, 130–31
    Creamy Cucumber and Dill, 132
    Fennel, Orange, and Arugula, 133
    Fresh Fruit and Spinach, with
        Orange-Poppy Seed Dressing, 138
    Insalata Caprese, 81
    Insalata Mista, 137
    Lemony Fennel, 136
    Liz's Pasta, 146–47

main-course, 128–29
Pepper Slaw, 140–41
Potato, with Green Beans and
    Tarragon, 149
Santa Fe Steak, with Lime-Cilantro
    Dressing, 144–45
and satiety, 127–28
side dish modular food list, 278–80
Tabbouleh, 148
Tangy Cole Slaw, 139
Thai Chicken, 142
Tuna and White Bean, 150–51
Volumetrics, 134–35
Zesty Tuna Pita, 124–25
Salmon, Poach-Roast, with Yogurt and
    Dill Sauce, 193
Salsa:
    Cherry Tomato, 240
    Mango, 88
    Tex-Mex, 78
salt, 265
sandwiches and wraps, 111–26
    All American Hamburger, 126
    Almond Chicken Salad Sandwich,
        114–15
    Asian Chicken, 122
    Buffalo Chicken, 120–21
    Chicken and Avocado Pita Pockets,
        123
    Cold-Cut Combo, 116
    Mediterranean Turkey, 117
    Open-Faced Roast Beef, 118
    Roasted Portobello, 119
    Zesty Tuna Salad Pita, 124–25

Santa Fe Steak Salad with Lime-
    Cilantro Dressing, 144–45
satiety, 6–7
    and carbohydrates, 11
    and energy density, 8
    feelings of, 40
    and fiber, 11
    and food labels, 7
    high-satiety food choices, 7
    and protein, 13
    and salads, 127–28
    and soups, 93–94
saturated fats, 14
sauces:
    condiments modular list, 290–91
    Lemon, 196
    Lemon Cream, 256–57
    Orange-Soy, 188–89
    Raspberry, 250–51
    Soy-Ginger Dipping, 82–83
    Tomato and Fresh Basil, 233
    Yogurt and Dill, 193
Sautéed Flounder with Lemon Sauce, 196
saving money, tips for, 266
seeds or nuts, toasted, 84
self-monitoring form, 50–55, 57
Sesame Mushroom Kebobs, 84
shellfish, see fish and shellfish
Shells, Broccoli and Tomato Stuffed,
    236
Shepherd's Pie, 184–85
Shrimp:
    Creole, 199
    Fried Rice, 200–201

Lemon Bruschetta, 80
    Paella Sencillo, 220
side dish modular food list, 278–80
Smashed Potatoes, 170
smoothies:
    B's Favorite, 90
    Tropical Island, 91
snacks, 72–73
    modular food list, 286–89
    see also appetizers and snacks
Snow Peas, Stir-Fried Beef with
    Tomatoes and, 181
soda/cola, 24
Sole Fillet and Vegetable Parcels, 197
soups, 93–109
    Asian Black Bean, 104
    Autumn Harvest Pumpkin, 96–97
    Cannellini Bean, 105
    Corn and Tomato Chowder, 95
    Creamy Broccoli, 98–99
    Curried Cauliflower, 100
    Gazpacho, 110
    Hearty Chicken and Vegetable, 108–9
    Lentil and Tomato, 106
    Minestrone, 102–3
    modular food list, 276–77
    Rustic Tomato, 101
    and satiety, 93–94
    Vegetarian Barley, 107
South of the Border Chicken Stew,
    208–9
Soy-Ginger Dipping Sauce, 82–83
Soy-Orange Sauce, Pork Chops with,
    188–89

Spaghetti with Tomato and Fresh Basil
    Sauce, 233
Spinach:
    and Fresh Fruit Salad with Orange-
        Poppy Seed Dressing, 138
    Penne with Olives and, 232
Spring Rolls, Asian, with Soy-Ginger
    Dipping Sauce, 82–83
Squash, Herbed Barley Stuffed, 171
Steak:
    Santa Fe Salad with Lime-Cilantro
        Dressing, 144–45
    Stir-Fried with Snow Peas and
        Tomatoes, 181
steps, counting, 44–48
stews:
    Classic Vegetarian Vegetable, 176–77
    Fiesta Fish, 202
    Nouveau Lamb, 186–87
    Old World Goulash, 182–83
    South of the Border Chicken, 208–9
stir-fries:
    Beef with Snow Peas and Tomatoes,
        181
    Crisp Vegetables, 166
    Green Beans, 164–65
    Turkey with Crunchy Vegetables, 211
Strawberry Trifle with Lemon Cream,
    256–57
Stuffed Mushrooms Florentine, 86–87
Stuffed Peppers, Bulgur and Vegetable,
    172–73
Stuffed Shells, Broccoli and Tomato, 236
sugars, decreased intake of, 29

T

Tabbouleh, 148
Tangy Cole Slaw, 139
tea, 21
Tex-Mex Salsa, 78
Thai Chicken Salad, 142
Tilapia, Baked, with Sautéed
    Vegetables, 194–95
Tofu Pad Thai, 167
tomatoes:
    and Broccoli Stuffed Shells, 236
    and Corn Chowder, 95
    and Herb Dressing, Nonfat, 143
    and Lentil Soup, 106
    Rustic Soup, 101
    Spaghetti with Fresh Basil Sauce and,
        233
    Stir-Fried Beef with Snow Peas and, 181
transfats, 14
Trifle, Strawberry, With Lemon Cream,
    256–57
Tropical Island Smoothie, 91
tuna:
    and Fruit Kebobs, Jenny's Caribbean,
        198
    and White Bean Salad, 150–51
    Zesty Salad Pita, 124–25
Turkey:
    Italian Spirals, 212
    Mediterranean Sandwich, 117
    -Pepperoni Pizza, 242
    Stir-Fried, with Crunchy Vegetables,
        211

V

vegetables, 155–77
  and Bulgur Stuffed Peppers, 172–73
  Charlie's Pasta Primavera, 228–29
  and Chicken Soup, Hearty, 108–9
  Classic Vegetarian Stew, 176–77
  Crisp Stir-Fried, 166
  Crunchy, Stir-Fried Turkey with, 211
  fiber in, 11
  Fillet of Sole with Parcels of, 197
  Garden-Fresh Pizza, 238
  Garlic-Roasted, 160–61
  Gazpacho, 110
  Herbed Barley Stuffed Squash, 171
  main-course salads, 128–29
  Minestrone, 102–3
  Minted Broccoli, 158–59
  New Potatoes with Peas, 168
  Oven-Roasted Potatoes, 169
  Party Platter, 74–75
  with pasta, 226
  Pilaf, 221
  as pizza toppings, 227
  Ratatouille, 162
  Risotto Primavera, 222–23
  Roasted Asparagus, 162
  in sandwiches, 112
  Sautéed, Baked Tilapia with, 194–95
  side dish modular food list, 278–80
  Smashed Potatoes, 170
  Stir-Fried Green Beans, 164–65
  Veggie-Stuffed Macaroni and Cheese,
    234–35
  water content of, 8
  in weight management, 156–57
vegetarian dishes, 155–57
  The Aristotle Pizza, 237
  Barley Soup, 107
  Chickpea Curry, 174
  Classic Vegetable Stew, 176–77
  Eggplant "Lasagna," 175
  Tofu Pad Thai, 167
Vinaigrette, Dijon, 152
Volumetrics, 2–3
  baseline week 0 in, 32–36
  food diary, 37, 38, 39
  principles of, 29
  success stories, 5, 31–32, 265
  Week 4-plus in, 53
  Weeks 1 to 4 in, 49–53
Volumetrics Eating Plan, 261–92
  customizing, 262–64
  focus of, 3
  meal comparisons, 4, 56, 62, 66, 75
  menus, 49, 269–72
  modular food lists, 273–92
  summary, 268
  tools for, 2–3
Volumetrics Salad, 134–35

W

water:
  calories in, 9, 24
  and carbohydrates, 11
  drinking, 11, 21

water (*cont.*)
   and energy density, 9
   foods rich in, 8, 10, 11
   in weight management, 29
weight management, 31–57
   behavioral challenges in, 48–49
   benefits of, 32
   body-mass index in, 34–36
   breakfast in, 59–61
   calcium in, 60
   calorie counting in, 27–28, 29
   cue control in, 49
   daily calorie needs in, 36–43
   daily energy requirements
     worksheet, 42, 43
   fiber in, 11–12, 29
   food diary in, 37, 38, 39
   habits established in, 48–49,
     266–67
   hunger in, 40
   personal goals tracked in, 32–34,
     51
   physical activity in, 29, 44–48
   plateaus in, 52
   and portion control, 25–26, 27, 226,
     243
   protein in, 12–13, 29, 179
   research in, 1–2
   satiety in, 6, 40
   self-monitoring in, 50–55, 57

   sustaining, 57
   testimonials on, 5, 31–32, 265
   tips for, 29
   vegetables in, 156–57
   Volumetrics Eating Plan for, 2–3;
     see also eating plan
   Volumetrics in, 29
   water in, 29
   weight loss goal, 34, 41, 48
   weight records in, 51–52, 55, 57
White Bean:
   Bruschetta, 79
   and Tuna Salad, 150–51
whole foods, fiber in, 12
wine, 24
women, energy requirements for, 42
wraps, *see* sandwiches and wraps

Y

Yogurt:
   Cheese, 89
   and Dill Sauce, Poach-Roast Salmon
     with, 193

Z

Zesty Tuna Salad Pita, 124–25

Conversion Chart

Use this chart to convert weight measures.

1 ounce	=	$\frac{1}{16}$ pound	=	28 grams
4 ounces	=	$\frac{1}{4}$ pound	=	112 grams
8 ounces	=	$\frac{1}{2}$ pound	=	224 grams
12 ounces	=	$\frac{3}{4}$ pound	=	336 grams
16 ounces	=	1 pound	=	448 grams

Use this chart to convert volume measures.

3 teaspoons	=	1	tablespoon		
		2	tablespoons	=	$\frac{1}{8}$ cup
		4	tablespoons	=	$\frac{1}{4}$ cup
		$5\frac{1}{3}$	tablespoons	=	$\frac{1}{3}$ cup
		8	tablespoons	=	$\frac{1}{2}$ cup
		12	tablespoons	=	$\frac{3}{4}$ cup
		16	tablespoons	=	1 cup
		1	pint	=	2 cups
		1	quart	=	4 cups